SpringerBriefs in Computer Science

SpringerBriefs present concise summaries of cutting-edge research and practical applications across a wide spectrum of fields. Featuring compact volumes of 50 to 125 pages, the series covers a range of content from professional to academic.

Typical topics might include:

- A timely report of state-of-the art analytical techniques
- A bridge between new research results, as published in journal articles, and a contextual literature review
- A snapshot of a hot or emerging topic
- An in-depth case study or clinical example
- A presentation of core concepts that students must understand in order to make independent contributions

Briefs allow authors to present their ideas and readers to absorb them with minimal time investment. Briefs will be published as part of Springer's eBook collection, with millions of users worldwide. In addition, Briefs will be available for individual print and electronic purchase. Briefs are characterized by fast, global electronic dissemination, standard publishing contracts, easy-to-use manuscript preparation and formatting guidelines, and expedited production schedules. We aim for publication 8–12 weeks after acceptance. Both solicited and unsolicited manuscripts are considered for publication in this series.

**Indexing: This series is indexed in Scopus, Ei-Compendex, and zbMATH **

Dietmar Dietrich

Artificial Intelligence: A Bridge Between Psychoanalysis and Neurology

The Psi-Organ in a Nutshell

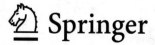

Dietmar Dietrich
Berlin, Germany

ISSN 2191-5768 ISSN 2191-5776 (electronic)
SpringerBriefs in Computer Science
ISBN 978-3-031-30367-8 ISBN 978-3-031-30368-5 (eBook)
https://doi.org/10.1007/978-3-031-30368-5

This Springer imprint is published by the registered company Springer Nature Switzerland AG
The registered company address is: Gewerbestrasse 11, 6330 Cham, Switzerland

With the support of
Klaus Doblhammer and Dorothee Dietrich

Foreword

Understanding the human mind has always been an intriguing question for scientists. This book presents, in a nutshell, the fundamental ideas of a model inspired by the layered functional concepts known from computer technology and computer science. It was back in 2000, while we were working on a joint invited article on the future of sensor and control networks as the nervous system of automation, that Dietmar Dietrich first discussed his idea with me. Since then, I have been following the evolution of this research work, being particularly intrigued by his approach to develop it, from the very beginning, in intense and sometimes painful discussions with psychoanalysts and neurologists.

This book is not meant to be a traditional textbook. Instead, it can serve as an excellent introduction to the problem of understanding and modelling the human mind—and to the problem of achieving artificial "intelligence" in general. It does not provide the details of a new kind of AI, but it increases awareness and understanding for the associated challenges. In that regard, it is a valuable supplementary text for advanced students or researchers in the field, notably not only in AI, but also (and perhaps primarily) in psychoanalytic and medical fields.

There is another aspect of the book that is perhaps not recognized immediately nor emphasized: It is a tale of how difficult real cross-discipline collaboration among engineering, natural sciences, humanities and philosophy is in real life—and how much it is needed at the same time to make significant progress. To me, having witnessed the hardships that Dietmar Dietrich has been facing since our first discussions, this slightly hidden aspect is perhaps the most appealing one.

January 2023

TU Wien, Vienna, Austria   Thilo Sauter

UWK, Krems, Austria

Preface

Although natural and social scientists today largely agree that the processes of the psyche are based on the nervous system, it is still difficult to grasp both as an entity. For me, this is already expressed by the fact that there is no term for such an entity. I argue that this entity must be understood as a unified organ, which is more than the sum of its physiological components, which leads to several important questions: How can we imagine the coupling between the two worlds, the world of the nervous system and the world of the psyche? Why is it so difficult for scientists to come up with a clear answer to these questions? As a computer scientist who spent almost his whole life trying to understand the bridge between *physics* and *information systems*, I know: The requirement for resilient answers is a holistic model of the unified structure of the *nervous system and* the *psyche*—let's call it the Ψ*-organ*—which satisfies scientific methods and laws. Thus, experiments and tests of psychology as well as psychoanalysis (and later even sociology to the same extent) are possible on a natural scientific basis via software simulations, from which it follows that their results also become objectively verifiable (in the understanding of natural science), independent of different schools. The dispute of the psychoanalytic schools could thus be finally reduced to clinical methods and principles. In the field of artificial intelligence, one would no longer be dependent solely on algorithms, but would have the human Ψ-organ, developed by psychoanalysts, as the basis for structural plans of intelligent machines. This, in turn, would have the effect of immensely improving complex systems, e.g., the safety functions of control systems for aircraft, drones, energy plants, etc. It must be understood that the simulation of the functional Ψ-organ makes its unconscious processes visible for the first time and this knowledge can be applied to machines.

The literature shows: To merge the descriptions of the psyche and the neuronal system has been a long-cherished goal of science [11; 12, p. 124; 14; 15, p. 251]. In Vienna, in 1999, the idea developed to use the findings of psychoanalysis from the perspective of natural science for this purpose. The project resulting from this idea was first known by the acronym ARS, and later replaced by the term SiMA. The publications and conference papers published on this subject—over 250 reviewed scientific publications and two books—, some of them highly controversial, are difficult to read because they presuppose knowledge of *computer technology, computer science, information theories, psychoanalysis* and also *neurology*. Even the most recently written book "Simulating the Mind II" (Shaker Verlag, 2021) did not solve this problem. In this book I tried to compile the findings of all SiMA research in as much detail as possible and with as much references as possible. Immediately after publication, cherished colleagues of mine recommended a more accessible overview/publication of this highly complex content, which would not require such a great extent of expertise in all mentioned research fields. It would dispense of too detailed explanations and, importantly, too detailed scientific justifications. *Put it in a nutshell!* This book is the result. It is intended to bring together experts from various disciplines and, above all, to motivate young people to engage in the topic.

In order to better understand certain critical points in the book, I must make one more crucial comment about axiomatics: The mapping of the largely hermeneutic descriptive language of psychoanalysis to the axiomatic descriptive language of natural sciences, like information theory, requires compromises. Concepts like *affect*, which is subject to several definitions in psychoanalysis, cannot be adopted directly and have to be defined unambiguously. In SiMA, for this reason, only the term *quota of affect* is defined. The use of term affect alone is consistently avoided. Appropriate compromises with other terms that are also difficult to define unambiguously are sought.

Berlin, Germany   Dietmar Dietrich

Acknowledgements

To merge the findings of computer science, neurology and psychoanalysis, requires a profound theoretical understanding of and research experience in these three scientific fields. One lifetime is not long enough to acquire this. Every author is thus confronted with the necessity of finding experts who are willing to delve into this complex subject, to discover its contradictions, to recognize open questions and to validate the conclusiveness of given explanations. In this sense, I owe a great deal to my wife Dorothee Dietrich, who, with her profound knowledge of psychoanalysis, but also with her basic knowledge of the natural sciences, understood very well how to dive into the different worlds, to give advice, and to discuss repeatedly upcoming contradictions. Likewise, my friend Klaus Doblhammer, a Viennese psychoanalyst and trained philosopher, contributed a great deal with his enormous knowledge of the crucial literature. He never tired of pointing out inconsistencies to me and recommending literature to deepen necessary aspects. In the same way, I must emphasize the help of my daughter-in-law Ama Dietrich, who supported me enormously with her scientific knowledge of medicine and her English proficiency, especially for her help with editing this manuscript, as well as my son Lars Dietrich, group analyst and psychoanalytic pedagogue. I owe much to their critical thinking and recommendations. I need not conceal that as a technician I find it difficult to express myself in ways that a diverse readership can comprehend.

Of course, I also have to thank all scientists who participated in the SiMA project, especially my former PhD students, who had worked intensively on this topic for 3–8 years. They provided critical and detailed feedback on my previous book "Simulating the Mind II". Their criticism initiated this book and thus made it possible in the first place. Writing it gave me great joy, because it also gave me a better understanding of how difficult it is to grasp SiMA's thought processes. If only I had had this knowledge earlier, I would have helped me making my lectures and seminars on this topic more accessible for my students.

Some of my colleagues and friends, who were not involved in SiMA but nevertheless read my previous books on this subject, were often frustrated with detailed technical descriptions, a dry writing style and too much scientific detail. I have to thank them for their critical statements and suggestions. Similarly, I would like to thank everyone else who had a closer look at this book and gave me good advice and helpful criticism. Here in particular, I would like to mention: Peter Baumann, Andreas Cieslik-Eichert, Volker Amaro Hartmann Cardelle, Christine Eichert, Horst Grimm, Henriette Löffler-Stastka, Johann August Schülein and Andreas Slemeyer.

Contents

1   **Introduction**   1

2   **Principles of Description**   3

3   **Functions and Their Behavior**   7

4   **Extended Mealy Theory**   11

5   **Information Systems of High Intelligence**   15

6   **World of Hardware: Neuroscience and More**   19

7   **World of Information: Psychoanalysis and More**   23

8   **The Ψ-Organ: A SiMA Model**   35

9   **Turing, Intelligence and the Self**   47
     9.1   The Turing and the Mirror Test   47
     9.2   Intelligence and Learning   49
     9.3   The Self   50

10   **Scientific Elaboration of Consciousness**   51

Literature (Cited in the Text)   53
     Several Bibliographic Notes   54

Index   55

Chapter 1
Introduction

We make our decisions with an organ that may strike us as the most uncanny of all the organs, and about which scientists in different fields argue most fiercely. Think of the trench warfare between neuroscientists, psychoanalysts, psychiatrists, and artificial intelligence scientists. Many of them are deeply absorbed in their own fields with no real discourse between them. Actually grotesque. And it is true, we make decisions with something that seems obscure, often contradictory. In the past, this "thinking apparatus" was appropriated by religion and philosophy. To this day, it seems sacrilegious and unthinkable for many to consider the soul and the spirit from the point of view of natural science.

In contrast, we as natural scientists would have to try to understand the world exactly the other way around: First we should precisely analyze the thing with which we think, decide and act, i.e. our spirit, our brain, our psychic or our mental apparatus, whatever we may call this thing, this "thinking apparatus", before we take a closer look at other processes. We should all be aware of the fact that only when we know our "thinking apparatus", with which we perceive the outside world, with which we interpret incoming information and try to reflect on it, are we in a position to better assess its limitations and its erroneous perceptions. Only then will we be able to make decisions more objectively, and only then will we be able to assess our potential, much lauded objectivity ourselves. Above all, only then can we understand what *objectivity* really means.

Up to now, religion and philosophy have taken over the task—of course from their point of view, via their logic—of explaining our mind, our soul, and our ability to think in such a way that we believed to be able to use this thing, this mental, this inner world as a *reference* for the outer world. But at least since thinkers like Spinoza expressed their doubts, we know that religions and philosophical considerations and their logic are based on fanciful ideas, which depend on the zeitgeist and often contradict scientific considerations and experiments [3]. So, if we want to work out a unified model of our body in the holistic sense, including the "thinking apparatus", the complete information system with all the inputs and outputs (afferents and

D. Dietrich, *Artificial Intelligence: A Bridge Between Psychoanalysis and Neurology*, SpringerBriefs in Computer Science, https://doi.org/10.1007/978-3-031-30368-5_1

efferents), we have to choose the scientific way of thinking. The alternative would be to bring together natural sciences and the humanities. Is this possible? How is the problem to be approached? Is there a solution at all?

In order to avoid misunderstandings, in order not to build up unnecessary resistance and pushback from the beginning, I will use the term Ψ-*organ* (Psi-organ). In the past, when I used terms like brain, nervous system, mental apparatus, or similar terms to represent this "thinking apparatus", at least one community always protested and accused me of using the wrong term or even neurological reductionism. For some, the term *brain* excludes the sensors. The term *mental apparatus* can be interpreted as a reduction to the psyche. With the term *nervous system* many cannot connect the psyche and so on. In contrast, the use of the term Ψ-*organ* implies several beneficial aspects at once. The word organ indicates that it is one unit like all other organs of the body. The lungs have the task of breathing. The heart has the task of pumping blood through the body. The Ψ-*organ* has the task of *processing, storing,* and *transferring information* in the human body. The term organ is intended to indicate that the sensory, actuator (afferent), neurological and psychological functions of this unit perform certain tasks that are characteristic of them. Ψ (Psi) shall stand for the fact that besides the concept models of information theory, the scientific model concepts of psychoanalysis are also taken as a basis. But why psychoanalysis in particular? From the point of view of a computer scientist, this is easy to explain: *Psychoanalysis is the only science that has, in a holistic sense, a unified, functional model of the psyche* (see the more detailed explanation in Chap. 3: *Functions and Their Behavior*), which, according to the *extended Mealy theory* of computer science (Chap. 4), can be merged with the neuroscientific ideas and does not lead to scientific contradictions. Behavior models of psychology are not suitable for functional simulations.

The reader realizes that the last sentences are no longer easy to understand. Correct! Basically, if one wants to understand the uniform model of the Ψ-*organ*, one must dive a little bit into the different worlds of the scientific thinking—the world of *neurology, psychoanalysis* as well as *information theory of computer technology*. The phrase "bathe me, but don't get me wet" in essence applies here. One has to accept getting wet a little, if one wishes to be bathed. Deep mathematical understanding, on the other hand, is not necessary. It is worth noting that logic, mathematics, graphics, etc. are only abstract tools and products (of the mind/ imagination). Natural sciences cannot exist without them. However, in order to gain a simple understanding of the various topics, this book will omit profound mathematic formulations. These can be found in the book *Simulating the Mind II* [6] or in the further literature I have suggested.

Chapter 2
Principles of Description

Mealy's extended theory (see Chap. 4) allows models of physics on the one hand and models of the information theory on the other hand to be merged. It represents a crucial tool for developing electronic building blocks (chips) of computers. In order to comprehend this theory, we must first understand: What are physics, chemistry, information technology (including information theory), neurology, physiology and psychoanalysis anyway? Physics is not the atom. Chemistry is not the connection between molecules. Neurology is not the neuron. But all these scientific subjects enable us to describe a something, an object, a process, or something completely abstract—for example the atom—in order to develop a model of this something, which we can use to help us understand it. Physics, chemistry, neurology, etc. are scientific subjects in which specific methods and laws have been developed over a long period of time in order to arrive at knowledge as objectively (and reflectively) as possible, and in order to be able to abstract and describe something clearly from the subject-specific point of view. In this context, this book only addresses the natural sciences, not the humanities or clinical fields. In clinical or humanities subjects other methods, ideas, and procedures are necessary. For this reason, I separate psycho-analysis, as Sigmund Freud did, into the clinical and the theoretical-scientific realms. He called the theoretical-scientific realm metapsychology. It is necessary for under-standing, for the model theory of the psyche, and for the ability to base clinical considerations on its well-founded ideas.

Starting from these considerations, one can look at a matter from the point of view of physics, but also from the point of view of chemistry. And: an information system, like a mechanical clock, can be described purely physically, but also from the point of view of information theory. Each area of natural science developed and continues to develop its specific methods and laws. The decisive factor in the natural sciences, as opposed to the humanities, is that there can be no contradictions in the descrip-tions within one topic or subject, but also between different subjects. Contradictions are to be seen in principle as challenges to science. They have to be solved. This is a critical point which non-natural scientists cannot simply accept, and to which I must

D. Dietrich, *Artificial Intelligence: A Bridge Between Psychoanalysis and Neurology*, SpringerBriefs in Computer Science, https://doi.org/10.1007/978-3-031-30368-5_2

therefore return later. But first I would like to address another critical point that I have often encountered in joint workshops and conferences of engineers and psychoanalysts: Psychoanalysis thrives on contradictions, just think of unconscious in contrast to the then performed conscious actions.

And there is one more issue I have to mention. Why do I, as an engineer and scientist of computer technology, not address the subject of mathematics in all the various subjects listed, such as physics, physiology, and information technology, when it is the central tool in the field of engineering?

In order to be able to discuss these two points more easily, I will begin with the subject of mathematics. One must consider that mathematics does not describe a "something", an object, or something that can be perceived or imagined. Mathematics is a tool, which is used in all other natural scientific areas, albeit with their specific methods, in order to be able to describe something abstractly and objectively. Mathematics originates from logic. We humans abstract forms, functions, behavior, processes, relationships, etc., define quantities, and connect and describe them using subject-specific methods including mathematics. In everyday life just as in all scientific subjects.

For this reason, I distinguish between the terms *proving* and *validating*. Mathematical algorithms are provable, i.e., their correctness is unambiguously verifiable. Why? Because they are abstracted axiomatically precisely and therefore can be formulated in such a way that the thought model is conclusive in itself. Imagine a simple triangle. Its shape or the ratio of the sides to its area can be clearly described. That is why the laws of the triangle can be proven. It looks different in physics, in neurology, or in information theory. It is not necessary to use Heisenberg's uncertainty principle. A triangle constructed of metal will never correspond to the pure mathematical model. To understand this, it is enough to remember how an architect takes a measurement of an apartment. Even if nowadays, laser measuring instruments are used rather than tape measures, the accuracy is still limited (in contrast to abstract—imaginary—shapes). So, in principle, it is not possible to prove the size of the area of a living space, it is only possible to validate it, that is, to check the accuracy with a certain proximity and probability. Mathematics, thus, helps in all subjects to abstract a something, to describe it, and even to determine the probable inaccuracy. However, if a mathematical formalism can be successfully applied in one subject, it does not mean that this formalism is also useful in another subjects. The experts of each scientific field have to validate via experiments whether they can apply the corresponding mathematical formalism in their specific subject, whether it is suitable.

With this, I return to the above-mentioned contradiction of explanations within, but also between different natural scientific areas. Correct, contradictions of explanations are in principle not allowed, because experiments are the basis of the natural sciences. And experiments do not contradict each other, only in their explanations, descriptions, or interpretations. One upholds their correctness until further experiments prove the opposite.

In order to better understand the consequences, one must take into account the history of craft guilds and the development of the different fields or trades. They lived and still live in different conceptual worlds, use their specific methods, and work out laws according to their needs. In each of their fields a different axiomatic is practiced. The definitions of terms are often made independently from other fields. If one wants to combine different fields of expertise today, e.g., by means of described models, the axiomatics must first be reconciled with each other. This is not only difficult in science, but also in the various industrial sectors and trades. National and international standardization bodies have to invest a lot of money in order to achieve this highly ambitious goal of information processing. It is important to keep this in mind: People from the various trades, such as electricians, plumbers, chimney sweeps, and bricklayers for example, have to sit down at the same table in standardization committees for the first time in centuries and jointly coordinate their terms and define (standardize) them uniformly, without the contradictions which have grown over centuries in the various sectors. Think of the psychological, ideological, and political resistance. However, without such standardization, electronic networks such as WLAN, Wi-Fi, fieldbuses, Internet of Things, etc. would not be feasible; without them, the coupling of the various components of the white and brown goods via the smart phone would not be possible. Information technology requires this coordination. When sensors (temperature sensors, switches, etc.) and actuators (motors, lights, etc.) are installed in a house, all the trades involved must have the same conceptual understanding of the terminology (axiomatic).

If one wants to unite the psyche with neurology in a common model, one cannot avoid first developing a common axiomatic for psychoanalysis and medicine, which must not contain any contradictions—similar to the problem in building automation, an area in which I served on many international committees, also in the realm of axiomatic, over a long period of time. For the SiMA project mentioned at the beginning, this was a decisive basic prerequisite, which took a great deal of time. You cannot, for example, discuss the terms 'feelings' or 'energy' if you have different understandings of the meaning of these terms. This contradicts any scientific way of thinking.

And why do considerations in the humanities, philosophy, or religion always lead to contradictions that cannot be resolved? They are based on different conceptualizations (including the axiomatic) and on logic which also depend on the zeitgeist and the culture. In other words, they are not based on scientific experiments. And that is also good. In addition to the axiomatic way of thinking, we also need the humanities way of thinking as well as the social contexts. We need culture. We must increasingly gain an understanding for their areas, for their meaning and purpose. However, their knowledge, their methods are not sufficient to develop natural scientific models. Their methods (e.g., how they define terms) partly contradict natural scientific procedures.

There is one point left open. I mentioned that I often heard from psychoanalysts at interdisciplinary workshops and conferences that psychoanalysis thrives on contradiction. That is true if you think about your feelings, or if you think about your own desires or ideas. All this is information that the psyche has to process. In electrical engineering, there is a subject called control engineering. It deals extensively with conflicting information. For example, which position should the wing flaps of an airplane take if different sensors do not deliver exactly the same information or even contradictory information? The first moon landing almost went wrong because the triple redundant central computer system worked according to the majority principle, and suddenly, two of the computers were "wrong" with respect to the third. So, the technology must also be able to deal with contradictory information. However, one must clearly distinguish where contradictions may occur and where they may not. Between the unambiguous designations (the axiomatic) of something (e.g., the functions of the psyche or those of a computer), there must not be any contradictions. On the contrary, one has to reckon with contradictory information passing through the functions. Contradictory information occurs permanently in technology as well as in psychoanalysis.

Chapter 3
Functions and Their Behavior

Computer technology gained momentum in the 1970s and 1980s as people increasingly understood how to abstract hardware circuits in a mathematically efficient way. A good example is the design method of the digital *Mealy machine.* The basis is to describe the electronic components, such as resistors, diodes, sensors, etc., in functions that exhibit specific behavior. But what do these abstract terms *function* and *behavior* actually mean?

The physician and cyberneticist Valentin Braitenberg [1] succeeded in making them tangible in his book *Vehicles,* rich in fantasy and spiced with a certain humor. He developed a playful thought model. Imagine a vehicle with two wheels driven by two independent motors. Figure 3.1 shows two identical vehicles. The difference lies solely in the connection of the two light sensors to the two drive motors that move the wheels. When a sensor is close to the light source, the motor rotates rapidly because the sensor is highly excited. In the left vehicle of Fig. 3.1, it is the right motor that is spinning fast. If the sensor is further away from the light source, which is the case for the left sensor, the motor connected to it (and thus the left wheel) moves slower. The result is that the vehicle moves away from the light source. The right vehicle behaves in the opposite way, it moves towards the light source.

Braitenberg defined the wheels, the motors, and the sensors as *functions* of the vehicle. They are subject to a *structure* (circuitry). Each function generates a specific *behavior.* In sum, depending on the structure of the functions in the vehicle, they determine a specific behavior. The *functions* and their *structure* are thus by definition the causers of a specific *behavior.*

The number of functions in the vehicles shown in Fig. 3.1 is limited to six (two motors, two sensors and two lines). The behavior of the vehicles is still easy to understand. In more advanced thought experiments, Braitenberg adds more sensors to the vehicle that respond to different physical effects and affect the motors differently. He shows how increasing complexity of the electrical circuitry makes the behavior of the vehicle more and more opaque. The causes of the movements are no longer easy to understand in their various dependencies.

D. Dietrich, *Artificial Intelligence: A Bridge Between Psychoanalysis and Neurology*, SpringerBriefs in Computer Science, https://doi.org/10.1007/978-3-031-30368-5_3

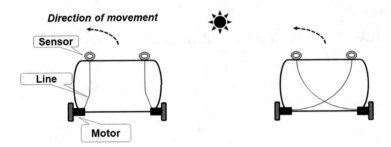

Fig. 3.1 Braitenberg Experiment

The conclusion Braitenberg drew from this is fundamental. If one considers systems with an increasing number of *functions* and increasing functional *structures*, their description becomes more difficult, but the functions and their structures remain manageable. Describing *behavior*, on the other hand, becomes disproportionately complicated, if not impossible. Let us consider the computer or the Ψ-organ. The complexity of the functions of a computer, its structure, is still well manageable to design, even the structures of the supercomputers of today. Understanding their behavior at all moments, on the other hand, is not only extremely difficult, but it is also often not feasible from an economic point of view. Not infrequently, we computer experts and computer scientists are faced with a puzzle.

And what about the Ψ-organ? As we will see, we are still able to design its functional structure. But to describe its behavior completely is definitely impossible. Who can describe the behavior of a human being in its completeness? The diversity is too great. That is the reason why psychology limits itself mainly to the description of behavioral phenomena. Psychoanalysis, on the other hand, takes a different approach, which I would like to compare with that of the computer engineer (and that of Braitenberg). From psychoanalytic observations and investigations, a functional model of the psyche was developed, the second topographical model of metapsychology. Sigmund Freud laid the foundation for this, and since then, as is usual in natural science, these findings have been improved, optimized, and refined. The first topographical model is a behavior model from the point of view of technological information theory. According to information theory, both model principles complement each other, since one describes the psyche from the point of view of *functions*, the other from the point of view of *behavior*. How does the information behave in the functions of the psyche? I will address all of this, including the topographical models, several times. It is essential.

In order to create a coherent picture, I have allowed myself to take a big mental step in the explanation, perhaps too big a step. I would like to insert therefore an "intermediate step". In the vehicles of Braitenberg one sees in Fig. 3.1 only functions to be described physically. However, if we address the computer and the Ψ-organ, we must also consider the functions of the information systems. What does this mean?

One must consider that every model of a motor, a diode, a resistor, or an electric line is by definition always the abstraction of a physical, real object. It is a representative of the real something, described by physical methods and laws. An information *function* is also an abstraction of something and it does something, it does something with information. For example, according to the information theory, the logic function 'AND' combines two binary input information to one binary output information. So, it combines information and generates new information via the logical 'AND' function. However, it is not described with physical methods and laws, but with purely informational ones. Accordingly, this statement is generally valid for all information functions, independent of whether it is about binary, ternary, decimal number systems, or the multi-value logic of the nerves (neurons). By the way, one can interchange the different number systems with each other, within certain limits. They are just different (interchangeable) description methods. This train of thought is not unimportant, since this interchangeability of the description methods is the precondition for being able to simulate objects of nature—like cars, airplanes, organs, or the psyche—with binary functioning computers although the nerves, from the view of information theory, are to be regarded as a system of the multi-value logic. That is, whether I program a computer to compute in the binary system, in the analog system, or even on the basis of multi-value logic as the nerves do, does not raise information technological concerns, only physical concerns, such as accuracy, speed, durability, and so on. All these, thus, ultimately lead to economic considerations, which I do not want to consider here.

Conclusion: If one wants to put together a uniformly described model of hardware and information functions, attention must be paid to how these two worlds, that of the hardware and that of information theory, can be described together as a whole. The critical point is mainly the exact description of the interface between these two worlds. This is precisely the topic of the next chapter.

Chapter 4
Extended Mealy Theory

George H. Mealy succeeded in 1955 in the development of the computation method of digital electronic circuits that is named after him. They are transferred into a two-layer model, whereby the lower layer contains the functions of the physical and the upper layer the functions of the information technological description method. It is a mathematical procedure, which one can only imagine abstractly. Mentally, one "tears" the real circuit into two blocks, into a physical and an information technology block (which, of course, is physically not possible). However, both blocks are connected to each other via a clearly (mathematically) defined interface (Fig. 4.1).

Just as one cannot really imagine the big bang of the universe, which Stephen Hawking derived via a singularity, so that time before the big bang by definition does not exist, the separation between a physical and an information theoretical description is to be regarded as an abstract, mathematical consideration. Our Ψ-organ is not designed to imagine such mathematical processes pictorially. However, we can learn to deal with it. This may also be the reason why it took decades for this theory to find its way into the curriculum in universities, even in the subject of electrical engineering. My experience as a university lecturer is that almost every student has difficulty grasping this separation of the physical and the information technological description. The term 'grasping' contains the physical or tangible, the pictorial, i.e., the physical imagination, which already puts us on the wrong track.

Back to the model of Fig. 4.1. What exactly is meant by the physical description of the lower layer? It means that all functions, quantities, and the carriers of the information are physically described there. For example, the functions in digital electronic circuits can be transistors, resistors, and diodes. The measured quantities can be voltages or currents and must be described physically. However, physics also means that time sequences must be taken into account. In digital technology that means: How long does a pulse take to pass a block of a digital circuit, or what is the delay time of a function? With reference to Fig. 4.1, this means that the information quantities which enter and leave the lower block (the information quantities a and h) are quantities which act on the human sensors or are resulting quantities of the

D. Dietrich, *Artificial Intelligence: A Bridge Between Psychoanalysis and Neurology*, SpringerBriefs in Computer Science, https://doi.org/10.1007/978-3-031-30368-5_4

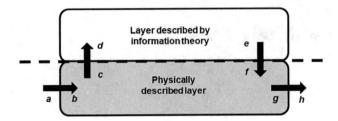

Fig. 4.1 Mealy model

muscles and glands and must therefore be described physically. The information quantities acting within the lower block (the information quantities b, c, f and g) on the other hand, are to be described by electrical methods, i.e., in terms of how large their voltage and current values are and how their time behavior is. If we switch to the upper block of Fig. 4.1, all quantities (the information quantities d and e) are described in purely information technological terms. Thus, the time in the upper block is to be seen purely as an information quantity. Physical aspects of time are not of interest here. The passage of all information through the functions of the upper layer is defined timelessly. If the information d in Fig. 4.1 is generated by the information c, the information e, which represents the result of the processing in the layer described in terms of information theory, is present at the output of the upper block at the same time and thus as quantity f at the lower block. Only the information processing of the upper block is of interest, i.e. how an information x is modified with an information y to a new information z in a corresponding function— let us give this function the name *XYZ*.

Not only were Mealy and his team able to prove, through experiments, that this model, the so-called Mealy machine, was not just a mathematical gimmick, but various scientists also developed modified principles. Today, every design language for the development of electronic hardware, including computer components, is based on the abstract Mealy model. No computer is conceivable without Mealy.

Equally important is a generalization, the *extended Mealy theory*. Imagine that several computers are to communicate with each other. The first standardized model of this kind was the ISO/OSI model (ISO: International Organization for Standardization; OSI: Open Systems Interconnection Model). The layer described in terms of information technology can be split up as required and the functions contained within it can be distributed according to their specific tasks. The layers are arranged hierarchically. Each column in Fig. 4.2 represents such an ISO/OSI model. The lowest layer (layer 1) is always the physically described layer that defines the connection to the other computers.

The original Mealy model (Fig. 4.1) was developed for the design of digital circuits, specifically, to obtain a holistic, functional model for the physical and information technological description. The generalization of this principle, or the extended Mealy theory, leads to models like the ISO/OSI model (Fig. 4.2) or the model of the Ψ-organ. But before the model of the Ψ-organ can be explained, we

Fig. 4.2 Coupling of
computers according to
ISO/OSI

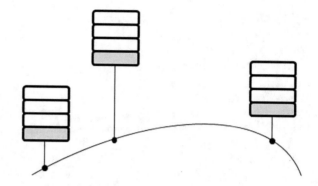

must first delve into the world of physical description—that is the hardware of the
Ψ-organ—and the world of information theory description.

Chapter 5
Information Systems of High Intelligence

If one uses terms like human, brain, psyche, artificial intelligence (AI), or nerves, the term intelligence inevitably comes into play. Therefore, when the first computers were developed, fantasies developed such as: Which computer and which micro-processor has the highest intelligence? Which hardware is the most intelligent? Which software? I will have to come back to this topic several times. But in order to avoid unfruitful discussions from the outset, I would like to anticipate two aspects at this point. First, there is no uniformly accepted definition of intelligence. Second, I distinguish between *active intelligence* and *structural intelligence*.

Structural intelligence is defined by its design. How intelligently, how optimally is the structure of an object designed? To what extent does a process behave efficiently for this reason alone? Braitenberg, whom I already mentioned, shows how a vehicle can be put in a position to drive in the figure of eight with minimal (intelligent) effort of an electronic circuit. A "sophisticated" *structural intelligence* is sufficient for this case. A few sensors, extremely cleverly connected information lines, and two motors fulfill the requirement.

This leads me directly to bees and other insects, which, unlike humans, have relatively few nerves (neurons), perhaps 10,000–100,000 [6, p. 102]. Humans, on the other hand, have far more than 10,000,000,000 nerves (neurons) [2, p. 331]. Nevertheless, these insects are enormously powerful because of the design of their nervous systems—because of their intelligent structural design. But I must leave out this kind of intelligence in my further remarks here. Their *active intelligence* is in no way to be compared with that of humans. In the following, I speak only of the *active intelligence*, which is achieved purely by the *processing, communication*, and *storage* of information. I will come back to this topic later.

I also want to leave out the hardware structures that form the basis. From the point of view of information theory, I may only be interested in one thing: Which information is processed and how. I would like to justify and explain this briefly.

The human Ψ-organ is the ideal system for the purpose of learning how such a high intelligence works. In comparison to other beings, it is possible to look at the

D. Dietrich, *Artificial Intelligence: A Bridge Between Psychoanalysis and Neurology*, SpringerBriefs in Computer Science, https://doi.org/10.1007/978-3-031-30368-5_5

Ψ-organ from the hardware point of view, specifically, the individual nerves and their connections to other nerves. On the other hand, it is also possible to approach a unified model from the perspective of the psyche, unlike in animals. For the human psyche, in contrast to other highly developed mammals, there is a scientifically developed functional model: the *second topographical model* or the *structural model* of *psychoanalysis*. For animals, there are largely only *behavior models* since one cannot work with them in the same way as with a human being. Animals cannot convey their unconscious ideas to us using verbal language. For the simulation of the Ψ-organ, however, we need a functional model (as Braitenberg (Fig. 1.1) almost playfully explains to the reader), which from the mathematical point of view corresponds to the neural model. We need the description of the functions of the psyche, in which the information is pre-conscious and conscious. But we also need the description of the functions in which the information is unconscious. Only the science of psychoanalysis offers us this theory.

If the hardware is the starting point in development, as a computer scientist, I call this approach a bottom-up method. If the starting point is the psyche, then I call it the top-down method. The reasoning is simple. With a material system in which information is processed, I always have a layer model with two or more functional layers in mind, according to my previous explanations about Mealy or the concept of ISO/OSI.

So, there is no reason not to describe the Ψ-organ as such a layer model, in which each layer has to perform specific tasks of information processing. The lowest (first) layer is always that of the hardware description, the uppermost layer must represent the psyche, described on the one hand via insights of the science of psychoanalysis, and on the other hand with the language of technical information theory. The connection between the different functional layers is represented solely by the information that passes through them.

The Ψ-organ is created by nature exclusively to control (direct) the human body, via information processes, as optimally as possible, and for all situations, to the extent that is possible. Its task is to preserve (maintain) the body in the long term. For this reason, physicians often speak of the nervous organ, i.e., a unified system with a specific function assigned to it, even though the organ is distributed throughout the entire body. This coincides with the ideas of us computer scientists when we think of distributed computer systems in machines or plants and develop models for them (e.g., the cloud principle). Each nerve has the ability to process and transmit information. From the point of view of computer science, a nerve can therefore by definition be regarded as a small biological computer—corresponding to the micro-computer, the heart of many of today's electronic systems. The complete nervous system, on the other hand, is thus by definition a network of many biological microcomputers, or the entire nervous system is a biological computer system. The many microcomputers are just not made of silicon, plastic, and sheet metal, but of living material. They do not work in a binary or analog way, but on the basis of threshold logic. They are therefore based on a different mathematical description method. From the point of view of information theory, however, it can be represented (modeled) in other, e.g. binary, structures.

Another short note: So far, I have for the most part used the term nerve. In science, especially in artificial intelligence, the term neuron is preferred. These terms are to be considered synonyms. There is no axiomatic distinction.

Chapter 6
World of Hardware: Neuroscience and More

There is sufficient literature on the functional structure and behavior of neurons. Therefore, the biochemical details can be studied in textbooks. That is not the subject of this book. Here, I would like to look at the neuron only from the point of view of information theory. This means, I will only roughly speak of specific aspects of the neuron.

A neuron is a cell with a nucleus, an axon, and dendrites. Think of the dendrites like the branches of a tree. They collect information from other neurons or from sensors via their ends. The carriers of the information are charged carriers (ions), which the dendrites conduct into the body of the cell. There they accumulate, leading to an increasing potential voltage. Above a certain threshold of potential voltage, the neuron "fires" (generates an impulse), discharging via the axon. Imagine the axon as a vermiform appendix of the neuron, at the end of which there is a branching, at the ends of which there are synapses. They dock to the bodies or dendrites of other neurons and release neurotransmitters (the discharging process) into a synaptic cleft, through which they "initiate" those neurons. The transmission of information from neurons to actuator cells such as muscles and glands occurs in the same way.

From the point of view of information technology, the neuron, and accordingly the entire neuronal network, is a complicated, nonlinear system for the *processing*, *transmission* and *storage of information*. Just as was done for analog and digital computers, scientists also tried to find well applicable mathematical formalisms for neural computers (one speaks of *neural networks*). But they are not as simple as the binary system of today's digital computers. Researchers abstracted in various ways, but the mathematically described approximations to living neurons and to living, grown structures of the human nervous system have not really been satisfactory so far. Let us be clear: Modeling such structures with more than 12,000,000,000 neurons, developing their structure solely according to the bottom-up method, i.e., understanding them building block by building block, is impossible. The corresponding problem was recognized relatively early in computer technology and computer science. Complex computer chip structures cannot be developed using the bottom-up method. This leads to errors and to suboptimal circuits, to "handicraft". Therefore, there has long been a consensus to develop electronic circuits using the top-down method. This is even more true for the analysis of complex circuits. More complicated information systems nowadays are modeled layer by layer, and in principle, one has to start a design (synthesis) with the highest layer. A supercomputer cannot be developed starting from transistors and resistors. You first have to understand what the requirements in general are, what functions are required in the highest layers, and how they should behave. Consequently, the lower layers are modeled solely according to the requirements of the upper layers and the given possibilities.

This leads me back to the extended theory of Mealy. Previous supercomputers were developed on the basis of binary logic and silicon. In the future, we will rely on the quantum computer. A rethinking for the higher functional layers is necessary only to the extent that the hardware becomes considerably more powerful with regard to information processing. The information processing laws and their methods remain the same for quantum computers. In other words, and this is a fundamental theorem to the extended Mealy theory: *The type of hardware and which description language is applied to the hardware should be independent of the information layer, and should follow the development of the information layer.*

Nature chose a different hardware than technology and did not end up with the simple analog, digital, or ternary method, but with the *threshold logic.* Nature can handle this very well. However, since we humans have mastered binary logic far better than threshold logic, we have had no choice but to use it until now. In terms of information processing, this has no effect on simulation experiments as long as the hardware layer fully satisfies the requirements of the information layer. As is always the case in natural sciences, the right application, the definition of the right boundary conditions (limitations), and the setting of the right parameters must ultimately always be decided by experiments. Consequently, this means: *The Ψ-organ can be simulated on the basis of our present binary computers. From the of information theory point of view, nothing speaks to the contrary.*

Let us return to the function of a neuron. I spoke about the fact that the neuron behaves strongly nonlinear. There are several reasons for this. First, the ability of charge transfer in the synaptic clefts depends strongly on substances like hormones. Second, the same applies to the threshold at which the neuron fires. The fact that neurons fire at a certain charge state also means that the actual information that is passed on is in the *pulse spacing (width).* Fast firing neurons mean a high value of information, slow firing neurons mean a low value. Thus, if information from different neurons flows into one neuron, the result is formed from the accumulating charge carriers and is thus in relation to the different pulse spacing of the firing neurons. It has been demonstrated that by combining the information of two neurons, one can generate a wide variety of mathematical functions such as addition, multiplication, exponential functions, and so on [6, p. 47]. This shows how enormously powerful, from an information processing point of view, neurons are in their nonlinear behavior, and that an artificial intelligence neural network abstraction is only a certain modest approximation of nature and certainly does not reflect its full capabilities.

This train of thought reveals another aspect. The neuron represents a function in two respects. First, from an electrical point of view, it is a hardware function whose behavior can be captured (described) by its quantities, its electrical pulse spacing, its physical energy etc. Second, it is an informational function whose information quantity can be described symbolically and can be derived from the electrical quantities. Perhaps by this example the (abstract) interface between the hardware layer and the information layer becomes somewhat clearer for explaining the extended Mealy theory. The symbolic quantities are directly related to the electrical quantities, described via the interface.

Still, another fundamental determination becomes apparent: The *coupling of the functions* represents the *structure* in a *functional model*, the *behavior* of the *functions* is described by their *information*.

Three more insights should be briefly explained before moving on to the next topic.

First, the *storage of information*: It represents a complex process in the Ψ-organ and must be modeled by several functional layers, like in a computer. However, these layers differ in part considerably from their technical counterpart, the technical computer.

To the lowest layer, the hardware [4]: The short-term memory can be imagined as feedback interneurons, corresponding to the flip-flop memory principle of electronic circuits. Long-term memory functions as the formation of synapses corresponding to ROMs of electronic circuits. However, the psyche's access to this storage of information, which can be described in hardware, does not take place via memory addresses like in the technical computer, but via associations. Therefore, parallel to the functional structure of the Ψ-organ, an additional multi-layered memory structure is to be considered, through which the psyche accesses the stored information.

Secondly, the differentiation between cerebrum and cerebellum: The Ψ-organ of the human being has evolved from a protracted development process. It is not for nothing that one speaks of the reptilian brain, the olfactory bulb, etc., each of which also evolved from ontogenetic processes. Consequently, the distinction between the individual brain parts, the cerebrum, and the cerebellum are essential with regard to their functions. However, we have to proceed according to the top-down method, which means to focus mainly on the structuring of the psyche. The description of the hardware and its structure must be left mainly to a team of neuroscientists.

Thirdly, the *hormonal system*: the hormonal system is part of the information system in the human body. We, scientists of information technology, speak in this case of a broadcast principle because the release of hormones is dispersed, and every part of the body that has the specific receiver can receive the hormones. These information channels are not considered here because the effects, from the point of view of information theory, would have made the development of the functional model very difficult. Furthermore, they are not considered crucial for the simulation of the psychoanalytic theories. Nevertheless, it is without question that the endocrine system must be taken into account in the long run of developing the Ψ-organ.

Chapter 7
World of Information: Psychoanalysis and More

According to Mealy, an information system is modeled according to a layer model in such a way that the hardware description takes place in the lower layer and the information technology description in the layer above. If the complexity of the information layer is considered high, it is subdivided into several layers (Fig. 4.2). This is also the case in SiMA. With regard to the Ψ-organ, a three-layer model with the following functional layers was chosen: Hardware (neural network), neurosymbolism, and psyche (Fig. 7.1).

I have already addressed the hardware; I would now like to turn to the layers above it. Directly above the hardware lies the layer of neurosymbolism, also called neurosymbolic layer. It represents something completely different from neural networks: the hardware-related description.

In the hardware layer, electrical signals originating from the eyes, nose, skin, muscles, urinary bladder, or ears are generated via light, odor, temperature, or pressure sensors, which are intermediately processed in neurons and propagated by them. Their pulse spacing is converted into information symbols in the interface to the neurosymbolic layer. In information theory, this process is called *coding*. It generates a vast amount of symbols, which are continuously received by the neurosymbolic layer. Furthermore, this layer not only processes the symbols in the interface, but it also creates an even much larger set of composite symbols itself. I would like to call all these symbols *representatives,* in the psychoanalytic sense of the term. They symbolize a something, like a smell, a sound, a haptic touch, a movement, an object like my finger, my hand, my arm, my cup, or my wife's cup. In the same sense, they symbolize physical states such as hot, cold, and bright. Thus, the ascending networks of the neurosymbolic layer enable humans, through *neurosymbolization*, to represent and, therefore, perceive the physical world in *abstract* forms and states (symbolized). I emphasize the term *abstract* because the neurosymbolic networks, starting from the interface to the hardware, summarize the information only *symbolically*, and, thus, only *symbolically* represent the reality, meaning in a very simplified way. So, what we see (mentally) is not the physical

D. Dietrich, *Artificial Intelligence: A Bridge Between Psychoanalysis and Neurology*, SpringerBriefs in Computer Science, https://doi.org/10.1007/978-3-031-30368-5_7

Fig. 7.1 The Ψ-organ as a
three-layer model
(cf. Figs. 4.1 and 4.2)

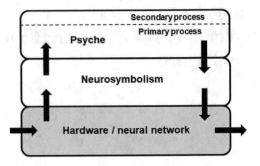

reality, but merely the *representatives* (information) created by our neurosymbolic layer of the many "somethings" that our sensors physically perceive. Formulated differently, we *abstract* smallest units like fingernails or fingertips and from them, we form the hand, then the arm, and finally the whole own body, of which every human being has his own imagination (his own "picture", his own *representative*). All these individual representatives are (constructed) abstractions of something, which are networked in our Ψ-organ in lists of objects. In tremendously large networks.

The terms 'abstraction' or 'constructed' are not negative. They are to be equated with 'manipulated' information. Perception means that a sense perception is brought into congruence with an inner representative via an abstraction, which results in a modification of the information. Here, congruence means both the information coming from outside and the inner information have a certain similarity. I would like to bring an example which, among others, illustrates a great advantage. The lowest neural layers in the eye calculate a much higher light contrast between optical transitions than the physical world in front of our eyes actually provides. *Thus, we see the physical reality sharper—with higher contrast—than it really is.* Similar efficient neural properties apply to other sensory organs.

What is my main point? Neurosymbolic networks have an enormous capability to describe nature, to map it, and to abstract it in such a way that the psyche can ultimately work with it in a uniform and highly efficient way on the basis of an almost inconceivably large number of the most diverse *representatives*, regardless of where in the body the representatives originate from (e.g., the ears, the intestines, the vestibular organ, or the muscle fibers), how they are composed and modified, and what states they represent. Neurosymbolism is the tool with which we can perceive our own body and everything outside our own body—but in an abstracted way. Therefore, psychoanalysis, from the point of view of information theory, even if it may sound strange at first, quite correctly differentiates between the *inner* and the *outer world*. The *inner world* is "within" the information space. The *outer world* is everything outside the *space of the representatives*. One's own physically describable body with all its sensors and neurons belongs, thus, to the *outer world*. Only the psyche and the layer that generates the symbols of *representatives* and converts them back into *electrical signals* is part of the *inner world*. The inner world can thus be equated with the world of information. It is an abstract, nothing physical. *The inner world is our world of imagination.*

Let us take an example of the *decoding* of symbolic representatives—the opposite process to *coding*. When our psyche instructs our arm to raise, our eyes to look to the left, or our heart to beat faster, these undifferentiated instructions must be broken down into ever finer details until finally each of the thousands of individual muscle fibers and glands are stimulated, resulting in a timed, uniform activation of the arm, the eyes, or the heart. And this happens in milliseconds. This is also the task of the neurosymbolic layer. From the point of view of information technology, this task can be called desymbolization.

So, the description of *neurosymbolization* has nothing to do with the description of the hardware of the neurons. And to avoid misunderstandings, it has just as little to do with the description of unconscious information. Psychoanalysis attributes unconscious, just like preconscious and conscious, information to the psyche alone, not to the layer in which representatives are formed (encoded) and split up again (decoded). The neurosymbolic layer between the hardware and the psyche is still completely unexplored. We know from technical communications engineering what might be going on in it, but extensive experiments and simulations with humans have yet to confirm these hypotheses. But why has no intensive scientific research been done yet? Anyone can visualize this. If one wants to approach this space of *neurosymbolization* from the hardware point of view, one first thinks of the 10,000,000,000 neurons. To derive a coding and decoding from this is hubris. In computer technology, engineers know this problem very well. Imagine a chip with billions of transistors, how can you understand it *without* a concrete circuit diagram, especially if you cannot measure currents and voltages? If one comes from "above", which means from the psyche, on the way to neurosymbolization one encounters the very large area of functions in which all information is available unconsciously (Fig. 7.1). How should one be able to work out the area below, the neurosymbolic layer, if one has not first explored and modeled the functions in which the information is unconsciously present? From this kind of reasoning, it is a must for computer engineers and computer scientists to proceed according to the top-down method, from which it follows that the first step of modelling is to develop the structure of the *psychic functions*. So, let us address this structure. After its model has been sufficiently simulated and, thus, validated, we can turn to the neurosymbolic layer as the next step, and then finally to the functional units of the hardware layer. Sigmund Freud recognized this very early on, although computer science with its technical information theories—especially Mealy's—did not exist at that time. This is highly fascinating to me as a computer scientist. Freud was way ahead of the times in terms of technical information theories.

Before I go into psychoanalysis in more detail, I would like to mention a very important physiological phenomenon, which also affects the neurosymbolic layer: perception. It was extensively explored by Jeff Hawkins [7], but only a few scientists really dealt with it intensively and comprehensively. Understandably so. The topic contradicts some traditional notions and especially previous fundamental technical teaching content. Moreover, perception requires knowledge from different scientific fields. Scientists of artificial intelligence or robotics mostly assume that the perception of an object should be thought of as in a camera system. The eye sees something and analyzes the image via specific methods. But this cannot be the case. Some things contradict this theory. How are nerves supposed to make analytical comparisons—similar to today's computers? More critically: Why is the number of nerve fibers leading *to* the eye much larger than the number of nerve fibers leading *from* the eye to the brain? For me, Jeff Hawkins promotes a theory that seems to be the most plausible from a scientific point of view. The Ψ-organ specifies, down to small details, what it wants to perceive in the now and compares these detailed specifications with the information flowing in from outside the body. Thus, even in the neuronal sense, the human being shows a willingness to see only what it expects to see. The approximate abstraction of the external (complete) object must already be stored in him. He must have once captured an approximation of it before and filed it away in his memories with a certain similarity.

Let us change the subject and come to the psyche (Fig. 7.1). In order to be able to simulate it and the neurosymbolic layer underneath it, the methods of the information theory in addition to the psychoanalytic methods are necessary. I have already summarized the essentials of the information theory in the preceding chapters. There is only one aspect I would like to emphasize again before I deal concretely with decisive psychoanalytic theories. It is often the cause of central misunderstandings. In technical fields, the findings from *behavioral* phenomena, mostly those described in psychology, are usually lumped together with *functional* correlations found in neuroscience and especially in psychoanalysis. And *artificial intelligence (AI)* today relies almost exclusively on behavioral phenomena from psychology and generally develops appropriate algorithms for this purpose. In the process, the terms *function* and *behavior* are often used in different manners. This must inevitably lead to senseless beer table discussions. I would like to avoid them. All used terms must be defined unambiguously, as always in natural science. I have worked in computer chip development and use the terms in this sense. They correspond to the considerations of Braitenberg. Let me explain this to create a common basis for further explanations.

AIBO ERS-7M§ from Sony is supposed to behave like a dog. The psychic functions of the Ψ-organ of a dog are not known. There are no corresponding structural concepts like there are in psychoanalysis. To what extent then does AIBO ERS-7M§ really correspond to a dog? I think the idea is that anyone is allowed to project his own fantasies into it. I do not think any technical developer of AIBO ERS-7M§ seriously asked himself what a (canine) Ψ-organ might look like in detail. Accordingly, the project idea of AIBO ERS-7M§ is diametrically opposed to that of SiMA. In SiMA, one indeed tries to understand the functional model of the human Ψ-organ—which means its functional structure—and to develop and simulate it in such a way that, as a result, the simulated agent exhibits validated human behavior and not just a few copied behavioral phenomena. Again, this is the reason that a *functional* model theory (in Braitenberg's sense) must form the basis. This is exactly the method of Mealy, but also of neurology. *This is the reason why only psychoanalysis can be considered.* No other psychological school besides psychoanalysis offers such a functional model, namely the second topographical model of psychoanalysis. It comprises the complete psyche and is made up of the three basic functions *Id, Ego,* and *Superego.*

With this in mind, we can take up the second major theme of this chapter: crucial theories of psychoanalysis. Again, I have to set limitations: I can only explain certain cornerstones of psychoanalytic theory, and clinical methods of psychoanalysis must be left out entirely. Thus, I must leave the subtleties of psychoanalytic knowledge to the experts, the scientifically active psychoanalysts. However, for those who are interested not only is there extensive scientific literature on this, but also extensive teaching material of various levels [8].

The enormous scientific advantage of psychoanalysis is that it has worked out a *functional* model of the psyche that can be *functionally* simulated. The basic principle corresponds to the *functional* model of neurology, the only difference that the functions in neurology are described neurophysiologically and those of the psyche psychologically. We also find this connection between the world which is to be described physically and the world which is to be described in terms of information technology in computer technology, where the *hardware* and *information functions* can be elegantly brought together via Mealy's theory. In psychoanalysis the functions *Id, Superego,* and *Ego* of the second topographical model are to be seen as the *generators* of our thinking and actions. All information perceived by sensors flows into them millions of times, 24 h a day. All the externally perceived information associate memories to find the respective optimal solution for an unbalanced homeostasis, for inner drive tensions, and for the resulting conflicts of manifold kinds that our psyche is confronted with, both for the current moment and for the future. The great flood of information is continuously processed in the psyche. The results of the decisions derived from this control our muscles and glands.

Opposite to the *functional structure model* is, as we formulate it in computer technology, the *behavior model* (often also, but not formally quite correctly, called data model). It consists of the descriptions of the properties of the information in the functions. These properties can be *unconscious, preconscious,* or *conscious.* All this information is always evaluated—psychoanalysts use the term *cathexis.* Not evaluated information, whether a thing or a process, does not exist. Not evaluated information—neutral information—is an idealized, "romantic" notion. In a human being everything triggers quota of affects and emotions. Everything!

In order to somewhat disentangle the complexity of the various processes in a task-specific manner, a further structuring of the psyche, in accordance with psychoanalysis, has been undertaken. Because of this reason, in SiMA the psyche is further subdivided into the *primary* and *secondary processes* (German psychoanalysts call it *Primär-* and *Sekundärvorgang,* see Fig. 7.1). If the three basic functions Id, Superego, and Ego, are subdivided into their subfunctions, those of the Id and Superego are in the primary process and those of the Ego are predominantly in the secondary process, only a few subfunctions of the Ego are in the primary process. All information in the primary process is unconscious. They cannot directly become conscious.

Fig. 7.2 The flow of information through the Ψ-organ *(L1: Hardware, L2: Neurosymbolism, L3: Psyche)*

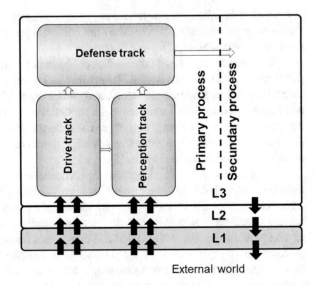

External world

In the secondary process it is more complicated. There, all information is pre-conscious or conscious. Preconscious information can become conscious when a sufficient amount of highly evaluated information is brought together. This can also happen when one mentally focuses on something in the here and now. In order for information to become conscious, the temporal *now* and the concurrent local *here* play a fundamental role.

In this somewhat complex issue, the question inevitably arises: How can the distinction between the primary and the secondary process be defined at all? Task-specifically! What do I mean by this? It seems appropriate to assign the functions in which information, which exclusively concern *thing representatives*, is processed to the primary process. In the secondary process, by contrast, *word representatives* are assigned to all thing representatives. The assignment of word representatives is a fundamental property and a necessity for objects or states to become conscious.

Let us have a closer look at the information flow through the psyche (Fig. 7.2), beginning with the perception track. Here, the symbols of the representatives, originating from the neurosymbolic layer (L2), are the input variables of the primary process. There are two perception possibilities. Perception of the body comprises the information of muscle activities, changes in temperature, pain sensations, and many other sensor values. Perception of the environment of the body receives input information through various channels such as visual, olfactory, or kinesthetic. According to classical psychoanalysis, all this information (*perceptual representatives*) is unconsciously and affectively (by quota of affects) evaluated in the psyche during the primary process. As I already mentioned, a neutral perception or handling of representatives does not exist.

Parallel to the above-mentioned two perception possibilities is the *drive track*. In it, one must again distinguish two information tracks (information processes)—that of self-preservation and that of the sexual drive. The process of self-preservation has input variables such as an imbalanced homeostasis of the body. The fundamental principle of the Ψ-organ intervenes here to satisfy the resulting drive desire: *The solution is sought in (evaluated) memories.* Which previous solution promises the most pleasure and the least unpleasure? Specifically, which actions stored in my memories promise to best satisfy my hunger, my thirst, or my urge to urinate? That this leads to contradictions is obvious, especially since the information of the perceptions, the long-term goals of the human being (in artificial intelligence: the agent) and not to mention the fantasies beyond that must also be taken into account.

The second track within the *drive track* (Fig. 7.2), the function of the sexual drive, is the basis for pleasure gain. The organic source are the hormones as well as sensory information from the mouth, the anus, and the sexual organs. They become drive representatives at the interface with the neurosymbolic layer. In addition, each drive representative associates the source of drive, an object of drive, an aim of drive, and a quota of affect. The emotions ultimately result from the various quota of affects, meaning from the evaluations of the symbolized drive representatives.

It is interesting to note that a connection between the *drive track* and the *perception track* occurs only in one direction. From the *drive track*, evaluated drive representatives are sent to the *perception track* and influence its activities, which of course can have a decisive influence on perceptions.

The primary process is not directly (consciously) accessible to humans. It has a completely different functional structure than that of the secondary process. It is the source (initiator) and thus the fundamental prerequisite for the functioning secondary process. It is the often misunderstood part of the psyche. Why? Because the primary process contains the most difficult to understand process flow. In it, contradictions continuously appear, for which the psyche has to find solutions by associating memories.

In order to understand this better, three methods of psychoanalytic description, which psychoanalysis calls points of view, have to be differentiated: the *topographical*, the *dynamic,* and the *economic method.* I have already spoken several times about the *topographical method*—the *functional structuring.* The *dynamic method* sheds light on the problem of highly conflicting information. As already mentioned, this applies to many areas, including technical ones, where conflicting information comes together. As psychoanalysis teaches us, however, the conflicting information problem is on the one hand extremely complex and on the other hand highly flexibly developed in the psyche. I must therefore come back to this subject. However, let us first talk about the third method, the *economic* method. In psychoanalysis, as I have mentioned several times, this means the *evaluation* of something. That is, the evaluation of something perceived by sensors, of stored information (memories), or of modified and newly formed information. The evaluation depends on many influencing factors and is decisive for all decisions in the Ψ-organ. Perceived, associated, or momentarily modified information is evaluated dependent, for example, on whether I am alone in the middle of the jungle, my children and grandchildren appear suddenly in thoughts, or whether I am comfortably reading a book at home while drinking a glass of wine.

The evaluation underlies the quota of affects of the different drive representatives and patterns of homeostasis. From these, emotions which can be subdivided into basic emotions like joy, anger, or fear, and into extended emotions like envy, greed, or pride are formed depending on where in the topographical structure, i.e. in which functions, they are generated.

Regarding evaluations, psychoanalysis refers to *psychic energy*, which misleads many to draw physical comparisons. This lures one onto a completely wrong track. Physical energy can flow, it is equal to matter. An evaluation, on the other hand, is a pure information quantity. It cannot flow. It cannot be described or treated like a physical quantity. For this reason, if psychoanalysis is considered under the aspect of natural science, as in the SiMA project, the term *psychic intensity* should be used instead of psychic energy. Accordingly, psychic intensity is the umbrella term for evaluations such as *quota of affects*, the different kinds of *emotions,* and feeling. Viewing evaluations as information variables also simplifies the understanding of the *defense system* of the psyche, which I will talk about in a moment.

In the primary process, functions associate information from memories. From this, modified and re-evaluated information is formed in order to gain as many possible solutions for decisions as possible. This unconscious information process is not subject to any temporal or causal logic. The primary process is exclusively about taking in the millions of incoming information (representatives and evaluations of something) from inside and outside of one's own body, deducing needs from them, and associating—from past memories—solutions that promise the greatest possible pleasure or the least possible unpleasure. I call this a great brainstorming of the functions of the *Id*, which the large network of *thing representatives* underlies. Perhaps some can guess the enormous power of its network with the help of their own dreams. The fantasies formed in them are far from any external reality. That distinguishes humans from (today's) machines. The information processes are subjective. Every human being compiles his own memories with his own evaluations and is thus shaped by his social environment. Conversely, every human being is part of his environment.

Essential functions of the psyche that are shaped by the social environment are the *Superego functions*, which belong to the primary process. Their tasks are *reactive* on the one hand and *proactive* on the other. The *reactive Superego* checks whether desires and proposals for action initiated via drive representatives violate internalized (social) rules such as: "You must not sleep with your mother.", "Be nice to each other!" or "Fear God!". The *proactive Superego* on the other hand initiates actions that promise high pleasure gain if the psychic intensity is high enough. Consider beliefs like "Every day a good deed." of boy scouts, or like "One should give alms to the poor." of religious people. Such demands must lead to contradictions in the psyche, just think of the unbalanced homeostasis.

There is yet another aspect: One of the outstanding abilities of humans is to develop strategies, to set rules, and to make plans for the future. But all of this can fiercely contradict momentary needs. In order to find the most acceptable solutions for this, the primary process, in addition to the enormous associative abilities of its memories, has another powerful tool at its disposal: the *defense*. Various functions of the primary process are assigned to the defense. It is very flexible and has numerous abilities to modify, shift, project, suppress, or even reverse information. And all this just to achieve one goal: to gain as much pleasure as possible or to have to put up with as little unpleasure as possible. I often have the following example in mind: While I am giving a lecture, I am thirsty and have no water with me, I also have to go to the toilet, on top of this, I associate a person in the auditorium with my son, ... and so on. And yet I am supposed to give a good lecture.

In other words: If we consider that 24 h a day a tremendously large amount of information from the most diverse sensors of the whole body flow in a person, which causes the most diverse needs, and that psyche, in addition this, must take into account the demands and objections of the superego, then perhaps it becomes clear why nature, over the course of human history, had to create the incredibly powerful defense (the so called *defense mechanism*). After all, it is important for the defense to only let the necessary and, above all, the survival-necessary solutions pass to the secondary process. The secondary process must be able to focus on the essential. And what is the essential anyway if one thinks of eating, hunting, loving, listening, talking, resting, writing, ...? The task of the secondary process—in contrast to the primary process—can only consist of weighing which of the proposed solutions of the primary process satisfy causal boundary conditions, which can be realized, and which then still promise the highest pleasure and the least unpleasure. The primary process thus associates as many proposed solutions as possible for conflict resolution without being restricted by boundary conditions such as causality or physical laws, and the secondary process investigates which of these are likely compatible with the external world and with one's own well-being and which are most likely to be reasonably implemented.

According to the current state of knowledge of brain research, in order to then decide on the right solution from the few selected proposals, a special function exists in the secondary process that can carry out two to three parallel trial actions (action simulations) before the final decision is made and muscles and glands of the body are actually activated.

This brings me back to the information property of becoming conscious. Examining causal relationships, simulating trial actions, or using our learned logic presupposes that words are assigned to the thing representatives during the transition from the primary to the secondary process. Thus, becoming conscious is only possible through language. However, it must be taken into account that humans can consciously concentrate on only very few aspects in the here and now. This in turn means that a large part of the processes does not take place consciously even in the secondary process. Much information is available preconsciously and can become conscious if sufficient intensity is supplied.

This leads to the question that brain researchers have been asking for a long time: Why do higher creatures have consciousness, while other animals do not? Above all, what are the basic requirements for having consciousness? What is the difference between *conscious information* and *consciousness*?

Today's consciousness research cannot yet answer many questions. But certain findings are relatively well-founded.

Let me take up the last question from above first. Its answer is the easiest for me. The term conscious signifies the property of an information. Consciousness is a property that the psyche can acquire.

Formulated somewhat differently: Consciousness presupposes that information in a person can become conscious. But consciousness also requires a *Self*, i.e. an 'image', better formulated: a self-concept. These images are continuously superimposed. There are several 'images', several 'concepts' of oneself, from which one conjures up the appropriate image in each situation, depending on the emotions and feeling in that moment. Old images, old self-schemas increasingly disappear in the background. I can no longer imagine how I felt as a child. I can only guess it.

According to Solms, I become aware of something when I develop a feeling about it. What does that mean? This refers to the hotly discussed topic of *'Symbol Grounding'* in artificial intelligence [10], which is viewed completely differently in psychoanalysis. Your proposed solution fits well into the model ideas of the Ψ-organ. I perceive all objects, everything physical, and all processes through the formation of evaluated representatives. If I focus my attention on my coffee cup, and thus establish a connection between my *Self* and the evaluated coffee cup, then and only then do I become aware of it. I see and feel it. It acquires the meaning 'my coffee cup'. That it is conscious to me, therefore, presupposes not only that I have a word assignment for this something, *but also a special feeling about it, and the reference to my momentary Self.*

This train of thought makes one thing particularly clear: the *Self* is multi-layered. If we imagine the Self simplified as stored images or short films, but not only optically, but rather as also as marked by the sense of smell or touch—or any part of the entire human sensory system—then it becomes clear that the system *Self* requires a tremendous amount of storage volume, i.e. an extremely high number of synapses in the Ψ-organ, which according to Damásio requires at least approximately 1,000,000,000 neurons. Worms, flies etc. can therefore never have consciousness, only more highly developed animals like monkeys, dogs, or cats. Thus, nature was able to introduce consciousness only after it had developed the appropriate conditions. On the one hand, these conditions consists of the size of the Ψ-organ (the high number of neurons and synapses). On the other hand, however, consciousness also presupposes—and this is my hypothesis—the elaborate structure of the psyche. For what purpose did nature create consciousness? Consciousness enables us to focus on the essentials, to see into the future and into the past, that is, to make long-term, logically reasonable plans and to evaluate them emotionally, despite the permanent activity of our millions of sensors and lively control mechanisms.

There is one more important aspect I have to mention, because it is important for the simulation of the Ψ-organ. Thanks to Eric Kandel, we know, from a scientifically validated point of view, how the long-term storage of information works via the formation of synapses [6, p. 207]. The storage process in the Ψ-organ as a whole can be viewed as multi-layered. On the lowest layer of a memory, meaning the hardware, the synapses are situated and can be thought of as the smallest unit of the memory cell. But how should we imagine different layers between this hardware and the psyche? They organize the access to the stored information of the synapses. Technical computers generally work address oriented. A piece of information is stored under a certain address and retrieved via it. The Ψ-organ, on the other hand, *associates* information. Contents are linked (listed) with other contents, which means, they are stored via other contents and retrieved via them. The degree to information is linked to each other is extremely high. An object is always linked to many other objects—we say, they are networked with them.

So, how does *forgetting* work? One thing is certain: simply forgetting is not possible. The subject is complex. If one recalls a piece of information from memory, it is combined with other networked information to form a new piece of information and can be evaluated via current emotions and stored in a modified way. This modified information is also networked with the originally associated information and the with other considered information, whereby an association of the old memory always influences the original evaluation through the new evaluation of the new information. The sentence: "I remember exactly this or that." is thus more a pipe dream than reality. The same applies to *objectivity* based on one's own memories. Objectivity is often mere wishful thinking and romanticism. Remembering is subject to an ongoing process of modification and evaluation. I call it insidious, creeping, indirect forgetting.

Regarding *total forgetting*: Synapses are degraded if they have not been activated by association for a very long time. However, since most associations happen unconsciously, one does not know oneself what one's primary process constantly recalls and thus keeps alive as memories. Let us take up an excellent example for all humans: The mother's breast has a central meaning for most people. For an infant it means everything. An associated representative is oral gratification. How could it be forgotten? For this reason, the defense system of the psyche has developed the mechanism to store these memories as *primal repressions* that only the primary process can access. The defense modifies the oral fantasies in such a way that the mother's breast is no longer consciously perceived in the adult. But it cannot be forgotten, it was too fundamental and is too strongly linked with many objects and states that promise pleasure.

I still owe one more remark. I mentioned that psychoanalysis today does not operate strictly axiomatically as natural science demands. This is especially evident when it comes to describing the mechanism of evaluation. Damásio [2] recognized this problem and therefore differentiates between affects, different emotions, and the feeling. In SiMA we had to go one step further because if this model is simulated, it has to be described mathematically, and that depends very much on how and in which functions the evaluation variables (quota of affects, emotions, basic emotions, extended emotions, and feeling) become active. Thus, affects are to be differentiated into individual, distinct values and must be described as scalars. Emotions, basic emotions, and extended emotions, by contrast, comprise multiple distinct values, i.e. scalars, which is why they are to be defined as vectors (as bundles of scalars). Feeling, on the other hand, is again an individual value in the secondary process and thus a scalar. All these evaluation variables, the scalars as well as the vectors, are unambiguously related and can be calculated accordingly.

Chapter 8
The Ψ-Organ: A SiMA Model

The Ψ-organ is an *information system* to which hardware description methods and description methods from the information point of view of can be assigned. Hence, it makes sense to apply the layer model according to *Mealy*. However, since the information variables of the psyche are the representatives and those of neurology are the electrical impulses, one must first ask the question: How should we imagine the transition of the *representatives* from the *electrical signals* of the nerves and, conversely, the transition of the *representatives* into *electrical impulses* which control the individual muscle fibers and glands? Mealy presupposes *unambiguous, noncontradictory* definitions for all the transitions in the model.

Let us have a look at Fig. 8.1. According to Mealy, the information in the hardware layer is described electrically, even in the lower half of the interface. The carriers of the information are the nerve impulses. The value of information is represented in each case by the spacing of the nerve impulses. In the information technology part, these electrical pulse spacings are interpreted as representatives—which means, they are described in the form of symbols and applied in information technology terms.

Symbol formation as a whole—not only the transition between the electrical and the symbolic description at the interface itself, but also the extended symbol formation—is a very extensive and complex process, simply because the representatives (symbols) are produced in an almost inconceivably large number. The idea therefore suggests itself to attribute the formation of all these symbols not only to a single interface as in Fig. 8.1, but to the interface plus the whole layer above the hardware. First, that means the symbols which are to be derived directly from the electrical pulses are formed in the interface itself, while a far greater number of symbol formation takes place in an additionally defined layer. Second, this means the block above the hardware layer, which is to be described in terms of information technology, is to be divided into two different layers L2 and L3. This was already mentioned in the previous chapter (Figs. 7.1 and 7.2). The layer L3 is the layer in which the psyche is described; the layer L2 below that, which is on top of the

D. Dietrich, *Artificial Intelligence: A Bridge Between Psychoanalysis and Neurology*, SpringerBriefs in Computer Science, https://doi.org/10.1007/978-3-031-30368-5_8

Fig. 8.1 Interface between the hardware layer and the information layer (see also Fig. 7.2)

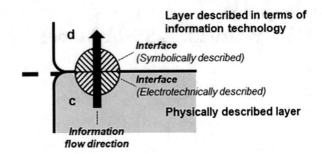

Now let me continue with the train of thought from above: I would like to try to

hardware layer L1, is consequently exclusively responsible for the formation (coding) of the symbols and the reconversion (decoding) of the symbols and sub-symbols. Therefore, this layer L2 is also called the layer of neurosymbolism. At the interface to the hardware, all symbols of the neurosymbolic layer, which have not been further divided into sub-symbols, are converted back into electrical signals.

Before I continue the train of thought on the coding and decoding of symbols, I must add something. It may sound confusing if I use the term symbol, and then also use the apparent synonym representative. We must always keep in mind that the layers L2 and L3 must be described via two methods, firstly by means of information and secondly by means of psychoanalytic theories. The psychoanalytic theories form the basis for describing the structure of the functions and the behavior of the psyche in models. The information technology description allows us to formulate a structure mathematically, in such a way that we can understand it as a unified, functional model. Both terms, *symbol* and *representative*, denote one and the same thing, each from the point of view of the respective scientific fields.

Now let me continue with the train of thought from above: I would like to try to describe more vividly the process of neurosymbolization, meaning the coding (representative formation) and the decoding (representative regression). If one imagines the coding of representatives as a hierarchical process, the "smallest" representatives are developed in the interface between the hardware and the neurosymbolic layer. From these, increasingly more and more composite representatives emerge. Decoding takes place in the reverse. Let us pick out one example. The smallest units which our eye can perceive are the irregularities of our fingernails. These perceptions are pieced together and abstracted in a representative as fingernail. Skin segments are added, then finger shapes, and in this manner we finally perceive our finger, our hand, our arm, our body, and also the clothes that cover it, again, always as new representatives. The respective representatives are therefore abstractions and thus involve the loss of details.

The decoding of the representatives takes place in the opposite direction. If, for example, a psyche's output function in the secondary process (Fig. 7.2) passes on the request to layer 2 to lift the arm, this representative is broken down into smaller and smaller representatives until the hardware finally knows exactly which muscle fiber has to be controlled in detail.

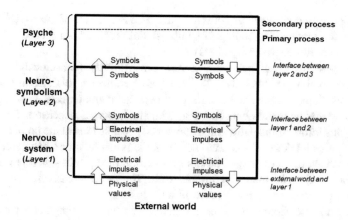

Fig. 8.2 Three-layer model

All these representatives are listed in us, that means they are information-technologically (symbolically) linked. Perhaps one understands now better why layer 2 is called *neurosymbolism*. On the one hand, it forms the transition to the hardware (the neural part), on the other hand, it prepares the information in the form of symbols for the *psyche*.

Figure 8.2 illustrates the whole process. It conveys that signals arriving from the external world (in the psychoanalytical sense), such as those from muscles, light, or the effects of force on the skin, are described in corresponding physical values such as lumens or newtons and then converted in the nervous system in the form of pulse spacing. In the neurosymbolic layer, the information transferred to layer 2 is only described symbolically.

Consequently, the principle information processing in the Ψ-organ takes place independent of the content of the information, independent of the origin, and independent of the target organ. This is interesting in the sense that one can no longer tell from the nerve signal where the information comes from and which sensors originally form the basis of them. The structures in the Ψ-organ thus play a prominent role in the interaction of the information. I immediately think of questions like:

– *Compared to an adult, which nerve structure of the Ψ-organ has a toddler formed?*
– *How does this develop to the point where the toddler eventually learns to speak and plan?*
– *What is innate, what is not? How do the structures change over the course of life?*
– *What is predetermined by the learning principles of the Ψ-organ?*

One can quickly get lost in thousands of questions if one goes into even just a little more detail. But let us stay with Fig. 8.2.

The neurosymbolic layer (layer 2) transfers the representatives produced in it to the psyche (layer 3) via the corresponding interface. Only in the psyche are they unconscious, preconscious, or conscious. Layer 2 is not part of the psyche; it only describes the production (coding of symbols) and reconversion (decoding of symbols) of the representatives (symbols).

Some neuroscientists believe that one can willfully (consciously), meaning starting from the psyche (layer 3), focus on specific nerves. According to the model, this would mean: The secondary process can communicate, via the primary process and via the neurosymbolic layer, with single nerves or sensors. So, also via unconscious information? How can that even be possible? From the point of view of information technology this is nonsense. What is possible is that one perceives the smallest sensor surfaces—e.g., sensors of a section of the skin—as representatives which the psyche can then play around with. The more intensively one trains or learns this process, the better the perception.

Something else becomes clear from Fig. 8.2: The computer engineers who mainly deal with systems described according to Mealy, i.e. which are based on a hardware *and* an abstract information system—such as computers—must always have the top-down design method in mind. The requirements of the top layer determine the tasks of the layers below, including those of the hardware. This makes it clear that in the modeling of the Ψ-organ, one must start with the description of the psyche (layer 3) before turning to detailed tasks of layer 2 or even layer 1. Without a doubt, one must never lose sight of the lower two layers when modeling layer 3, which is why one always includes even a rough abstraction of them in the modeling and assign them dummies, at least as placeholders (see layers 2 and 1 in Fig. 7.2).

In information technology, another method has been developed for top-down design: In addition to the layers, *levels* are introduced (the abbreviations L1, L2, and L3 are for layers, and Le1, Le2, ... are for levels). What is the meaning of this? The various layers in the layer model are assigned different tasks, like in the Mealy model for example. The lower layer describes the hardware of the information system, the layers above the information technology part. These are two completely different tasks. If the individual layers are difficult to understand, as in the Ψ-organ, each layer can be either subdivided into further sublayers (as explained in Chap. 4), or, if this cause problems, each layer can be described in levels. However, these single levels only represent different abstractions of the respective layer. According to SiMA, the lowest level of layer 3 is level 1, which represents all details (the lowest abstraction). The topmost level of layer 3 is level 5, i.e. the one with the greatest possible abstraction and thus the representation with the least details.

Figure 8.3 is intended to illustrate this. Only a few levels are indicated for layer 2, five levels were defined in SiMA for layer 3. As I already mentioned, Level 5—the uppermost level of layer 3—is reduced to one function, the psyche. In level 4, the psyche is broken down to its three functions *Id*, *Superego*, and *Ego*. In level 3, these three functions are described in a differentiated way again, and so on, until, finally, 32 mental functions which can be described individually are obtained in the lowest level 1 of the psyche (layer 3) in the SiMA-model. Breaking them down further is not necessary. They can be defined independently of each other. Their dependencies on the overall system can be described solely by their various input and output variables as well as parameter variables.

Fig. 8.3 Layer and level
model as a 3D model

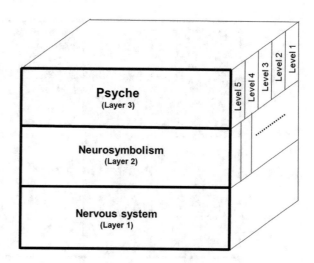

Thus, level 1 of layer 3 is the level to which the lowest degree of abstraction is attributed and at the same time, allows all *structural interdependencies* of the individual functions in the overall structure of the psyche to become visible in detail.

To date, the levels of layer 2 have not been explicitly developed, since according to the top-down principle, layer 3 must first have been satisfactorily, accurately modelled over many experiments before one attempts this major task.

Since modeling levels constitutes a software-technical method, the level model is not used in layer 1. For the hardware description, there are physical (neurological, electrotechnical, etc.) methods available.

I would therefore now like to solely focus on the essential features of layer 3 (the psyche), specifically on levels 3 to 1. Figure 7.2 shows an approximation of level 3, only that the transition between the primary and secondary process as well as the entire secondary process are not yet considered functionally differentiated. If one inserts the appropriate functions, one gets as a result Fig. 8.4. It shows the complete model, in which layers 1 and 2 (L1 and L2) are only considered as black boxes, while Layer 3 (L3, the psyche) is already differentiated into individual functions (here in level 3, designated as tracks).

The input variables (I1 and I2) of the Ψ-organ model, i.e., the information from the outside world, are the arrows at the bottom left of Fig. 8.4. The sensors send electrical signals which are neurally processed and transmitted in layer 1. The representatives, which are subdivided into two channels and are thus available as input variables in the *primary process* of layer 3, are formed in the interface between layer 2 and 3 and formed in layer 2 itself. Psychoanalytic theory asserts that there must be two channels. One channel leads to the drive track; the origin is hormones. The other information flow leads to the perception track, and has its origin in the sensors of the muscles, the skin, the eyes, and the pain sensors.

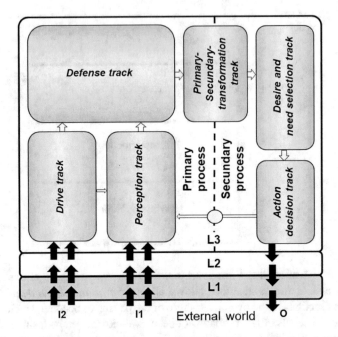

Fig. 8.4 The Ψ-organ in level 3 (psyche = layer 3 (L3) shown in tracks; layer 2 (L2) and layer 1 (L1) as black boxes; Input 1 (I1) and 2 (I2); Output (O))

Fundamentally, according to classical psychoanalytic theory, the representatives in the primary process are unconscious, meaning this process is *completely* unconscious.

Let us go into a little more detail and first talk about the perception track. It can be subdivided into the environment track and the body perception track, which is why input channel 1 (I1) in Fig. 8.4 is subdivided in two channels (see the two input arrows for I1). The task of the perception track is very complex and it is likely to be far more complicated than the simplified assumption in SiMA so far. Jeff Hawkins [7] developed, based on the findings of brain researchers, the theory that the brain always determines what, for example, the eye should see, which explains why more nerves lead from the brain to the eye than vice versa. This means that, on the one hand, an association is made about which *thing representatives* are a possibility for what the eye should see, and, on the other hand, which ones match, with a high probability, what the eye is actually seeing in the moment. These processes take place according to an immensely abstract sequential process that corresponds to the top-down principle. The highest representative level is the completely abstracted thing representative, which then gets broken down to smaller and smaller thing representatives until, finally, the lowest neural level of the eye—the cones and rods—"knows" what it should see in detail.

Of course, this does not only apply to the eye, but to all sensory perception units of the human body. The complete process of perception only partly takes place in the perceptual track of the primary process; presumably, it is for the most part a process of layer 2. The more precise division must be the task of further scientific investigations, which can be based on the simulation of the Ψ-organ model.

Figure 8.4 also shows an arrow from the drive track to the perception track. This means that quota of affects and emotions of the drive track influence the perception track by prioritizing thing representatives that promise a higher pleasure. Thus, what is associated and what is not depends very much on our affect and emotion state. This makes clear that "objective perception" is a glorified notion, or, as I mentioned before, a romanticized ideal of our abilities.

Primal repression also takes place in the perception track. I already mentioned the maternal breast. For a baby, it is probably the most important thing, and it is profoundly imprinted on our imaginations. It is therefore constantly unconsciously "remembered" and can, thus, never be forgotten. It would be more than annoying if this memory were to become conscious all the time. Therefore, it is *primally repressed* and can never—thanks to the defense—directly reach the secondary process via the defense.

One more function of the perception track is worth emphasizing here: the function for discharging *psychic intensity* (or *psychic energy* in psychoanalysis). Pleasure gain can be achieved not only via the *drive track*, but also via the *perception track*, namely via a mental sense of achievement, if the *drive track* creates the prerequisite for this. When I write this little book, I achieve a goal that I have set for myself, and the sentences that are formed in the process, which seem successful to me, generate a satisfaction via the *drive track* that is not inferior to the satisfaction, e.g., from eating a schnitzel. On the contrary, the satisfaction can be greater. In psychoanalysis one speaks of *sublimation* (the displacement of an aim of drive to a higher socially valued one). The ability to use it is considered a sign of maturity in a person. A precondition of a sublimation is a *neutralization* of the *psychic intensity* in the drive track. But how does the relationship between the corresponding tracks or functions work?

This brings us to the principles and structure of the drive track. Its information flow at input 2 (I2) consists of the quota of affects of the *sexual drive representatives* on the one hand and the quota of affects of the *self-preservation drive representatives* on the other hand. This explains why two channels are also drawn for I2 in Fig. 8.4.

Self-preservation drive representatives feed on an imbalanced homeostasis. Thus, one of the first tasks of the drive track is to associate solutions from memories to satisfy the resulting drive wishes. The task is to find out which associated actions, based on their evaluations (especially past evaluations), promise to best satisfy my hunger, my thirst, or my urge to urinate. What promises me the greatest pleasure and the least unpleasure in my subsequent action? That this leads to contradictions is logical, especially when one considers his or her short-term and long-term goals at the same time, not to mention when one factors in his or her other fantasies, or different events occurring all around.

The other information flow of I2, namely that of the *sexual drive representatives*, creates pleasure gain on the one hand, but on the other hand it is also supposed to guarantee genital reproduction. Hormones are to be seen as the organic origin of this information flow. They form drive representatives, to each of which—as mentioned before—a *drive source*, a *drive aim*, a *drive object,* and a *quota of affect* is assigned (associated). They decisively shape the individual character of a person. From the evaluations of the symbolized drive representatives—the various quota of affects— *emotions* are ultimately determined, from which *feeling* emerges in the secondary process.

Let us return to the important subject of *sublimation*. At the end of the drive track, a function which has the task of neutralizing the *psychic intensity* is formed. This is also called desexualization in psychoanalysis. It can reduce the *evaluations* of passing information, i.e. quota of affect representatives, and assign them to other functions in the *perception track*, but especially to functions of the defense and the secondary process. This process is an *evaluative* displacement. Caution. In psychoanalysis it is referred to as a 'psychic energy flow'. This cannot be accepted from Mealy's point of view, i.e. from the point of view of natural science, because *evaluations are information*, not matter. Information cannot flow. Only the carriers of the information consist of matter, and they are exclusively part of layer 1.

In the previous chapter, I spoke about the *evaluation mechanism* of the psyche. *Psychic intensity* is the umbrella term of all evaluation variables. In SiMA, a distinction is made between (1) the *quota of affects*, (2) the different types of *emotions* such as *basic* and *extended emotions*, and (3) the *feeling*. The *quota of affects* are formed in the first functions of the drive track (Fig. 8.4). The basic and the extended emotions are formed over the course of information shaping in the drive track and depend on many influences, of course also on individual parameters. Feeling, an evaluation variable that only comes into play in the secondary process, is calculated in a primary-secondary transformation track function.

There is no question that these extensions of psychoanalytic theories and the consequent more precise differentiations of the evaluation processes must not contradict the current findings of psychoanalysis. Rather, they must fit seamlessly into the overall picture of psychoanalysis. There is also no doubt that the evaluation mechanism of the psyche in detail is an extremely complex process, the modeling of which is still in its infancy and accordingly still requires many experiments until one can arrive at a robust model. According to the current state of knowledge based on Lurija [9], Panksepp, Solms [13] or Damásio [2], one can differentiate between quota of affects—such as those of perception (= body and environment perception) and those of drive representatives (= libidinous and aggressive drives)—from which the emotion vector is then formed, with its scalars pleasure, unpleasure, sum of libidinous and aggressive drive representatives, etc. From this emotion vector, the basic emotion vector—with its scalars joy, anger, fear, sadness, happiness saturation, exhilaration, etc.—can be derived. However, I suspect that these detailed definitions are, axiomatically speaking, not yet sufficiently aligned with each other. This is also because extensive simulation experiments—a core principle of natural science—are still missing. One must also consider that all these definitions belong to the zeitgeist of today and must accordingly be extensively discussed by the respective societies.

Let me come to the defense track in Fig. 8.4, which entails the Superego function. We have to differentiate between the *reactive* and the *proactive Superego* function. The reactive Superego checks whether information that is to be passed on violates internalized rules. For this purpose, information regarding a drive demand and/or a perception of the external world is utilized, which is based on evaluations by quota of affects, various emotions, and, above all, target specifications of the Superego function. The massive combination of all the evaluated information can hardly lead to a yes/no decision. But it is the task of the defense functions to find solutions in every case and for any conflict whatsoever, and thus bring about a decision. The defense has extensive techniques at its disposal for this purpose. Before I go into this, however, first a word on the proactive superego. At the entrance of this function, there is a subfunction where all emotions are merged. The basic emotions that can generate extensive associations also flow in here. Very easily, they can pop up in harsh contradiction to other concurrent cognitive ideas. This is often used as a striking example: "Do a good deed daily!". If this is sufficiently internalized, then compliance generates a pleasure gain.

With the knowledge that not only the most diverse information of the perception and the drive track with their various needs, but also the Superego continuously generate manifold conflicts, it perhaps becomes obvious that the task of the defense is enormous. I already spoke in detail about its manifold techniques, from displacement, modifications, projection, denial through to the reversal of information into the opposite. As an example, I would like to talk about a well-known and obvious trick of the defense, so that its abilities can be better understood.

A baby has the reflex to suck when it touches its mother's breast. It learns intuitively that hunger and breast belong together. The two thing representatives, the activity of sucking and the gain of pleasure, are symbolically associatively linked. If the breast, hunger, or sucking is perceived or remembered, the other representatives are associated with it. But with increasing age this would lead to confusion. Such associations have to be repressed—usually initiated by the process of weaning—in men as well as in women. Psychoanalysis speaks in such a case of a *primal repression*, as I already pointed out. The repressed content is thus no longer consciously remembered. Unconsciously, the breast stands for the greatest possible oral satisfaction of the human being. How does this happen? If the child is weaned, the breast, the greatest possible satisfaction, is withdrawn from the child. Psychological stress, and thus a tremendous unpleasure, cannot be avoided. The child has to turn to another object to cope with the pain. This is called *displacement*, which starts at the age of 2–3 years when the child's *consciousness* awakens. Of course, the origin of the process must never become conscious. We must deny it. The memory does not erase itself either because the representatives associated with it are permanently activated from the beginning. Fervent smoking, drinking, or gambling are thereby almost self-explanatory.

According to Fig. 8.4, the largest part of the primary process is explained with the drive, perception, and defense tracks. According to the model of the Ψ-organ, it contains 19 psychical functions. Four other functions are defined as transitional functions, three of which form the *primary-secondary transformation track*. On the one hand, this track is the function in which the feeling is determined from the quota of affects and the various emotions, which are used for the evaluation of all word representatives of the secondary process. On the other hand, it is the two functions that process the information from the perception and the drive representatives for the secondary process.

The fourth function between the primary and secondary process is a feedback function. In Fig. 8.4, this is shown as an arrow from the action decision track (in the secondary process) to the perception track (in the primary process) and belongs to the primary-secondary transformation track. In this manner, the representative parts of the secondary process come back directly into the primary process. This is the only way to explain unconscious fantasies. But how can one imagine the process more precisely?

In the feedback function, preconscious information is first split into thing and word representatives, and the thing representatives are fed back into the primary process. These thing representatives can trigger enormous avalanches of associations in the primary process. Enormous because, as already mentioned, they are networked there in tremendously large lists, which can be fueled by the emotions of the drive track. The feedback from the secondary process to the primary process can lead to imaginative cognitive performances in this way.

Feedback is of fundamental importance in technology. Norbert Wiener has already impressively proved that nature, just like automation technology, would not be able to cope without feedback. How does the process work when we pick up an egg, or walk, or climb stairs? Without the feedback of information on what our muscles are doing in this exact moment, how tightly we are gripping, how we are moving our fingers, our hand, our leg, and our foot, we could never achieve the precision of our movement sequences. It took roboticists a long time before their machines could grasp an egg. And our hands can still do it more elegantly. Like feedback in the physical world, feedback in the information world, such as the psyche, can have powerful effects. However, feedback is not without its problems. If it is set incorrectly, it can lead to increasing oscillations of the movement. Dangerous situations can arise. In the SiMA model, feedback has so far been largely avoided for this reason, but if the model is to be developed in greater detail and more precisely, this issue must be dealt with intensively.

Let us turn to the *secondary process*. Three main characteristics distinguish it: First, word representatives are assigned to thing representatives. Second, the representatives are subjected to a causality test, and third, it is checked whether these representatives can furthermore be brought into harmony with the external reality. That means, the past is seen as a memory, the future as a possibility of how it could happen. In other words, it is only through the secondary process that a person is enabled to make plans, to reflect on the past and think logically, to conduct mathematical proofs, and so on. And beyond all these activities, there are enormous abilities which distinguish humans from other living beings. Let us consider the aspect of making plans. It implies that in the secondary process, it can be planned to get from point A, through points B, C, etc., to point Z. In SiMA, we call these processes *acts*. For example, I may have a desire to get a coffee, which requires the following abstract act: Point *A* in this case is my place in front of the computer, from there I go to point *B*, which would be the door of my room, then through the corridor etc., until I reach point *Z*, the place where the longed-for coffee machine is. In my act (plan) all these different places are connected with memories—of optical kind, of floor textures, of sounds or smells—which become conscious only if the reality does not correspond to the unconscious associated memories, or if I for some reason concentrate on these places. Otherwise, the course of the act usually remains largely unconscious, which makes remembering "hardly" possible. I use the term "hardly" purposefully, because associations can unconsciously be awakened by external objects or processes, which are never consciously, and therefore never actually, "forgotten".

But what path does the information take in the secondary process to generate such *acts*? On the one hand, drive wishes (= drive representatives), with various associations, that could pass the defense reach the secondary process from the primary-secondary transformation track (Fig. 8.4). The amount and the kind of associations depend on the provided psychic intensity, which means on the evaluation mechanism. On the other hand, the formed word representatives, evaluated through feelings, are fed into the *desire and need selection track*. Since the *defense track* of the primary process already withholds the overwhelming majority of information, the desire and need selection track does not have too many decisions to make. But the possibilities are subjected to strict criteria, such as whether they satisfy the "external" reality or the causality criteria. In addition, there is an interesting point that Mark Solms reports on several times, namely that the psyche performs *trial actions*. And trial actions, for a technician, are nothing more than simulations, which, in the SiMA project, is how we test and validate the model itself. According to Solms, two or three simulation experiments can run in parallel. They probably take place in a highly abstracted manner and in the very short timespan of milliseconds. In any case, they remain unconscious, as they would extremely interfere with conscious processes. However, there is still a lot of research—and especially simulations—to be done in this area. The hypotheses are not yet supported to a sufficient degree.

The goal of the simulations in the secondary process is to find out which actions promise the highest pleasure and the least unpleasure, not only in the short term, but also in the medium, and especially in the long term. The *action decision track* (Fig. 8.4) then ultimately decides which action will be performed not only mentally but also physiologically. This information is additionally fed to the primary process, though reduced to the emotionally evaluated thing representatives.

Going into the details of the 32 functions of layer 3 (psyche) in level 1 that have been defined in SiMA so far would let the description in this little book get out of hand. Most readers would be bored by these details. Those who are interested, however, will find it in Dietrich [6] or corresponding publications of different scientists. Just a note to add: In the Ψ-organ 19 functions are assigned to the primary

Fig. 8.5 The Ψ-organ
shown in three layers *(layer
3 (L3) in level 1 with all the
individual functions
(32 defined so far)
highlighted separately)*

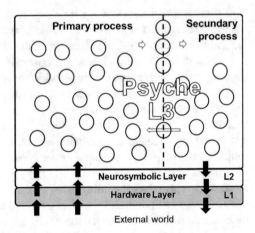

process of the psyche in level 1, 9 to the secondary process, and 4 between the
primary and secondary processes. This is shown in a strongly abstracted form—
without the described functional structure of the psyche—in Fig. 8.5. As before,
layers 1 and 2 are always indicated only as black boxes.

Chapter 9
Turing, Intelligence and the Self

In order to better grasp the scope of the model of the Ψ-organ, I would like to address three more topics. In my opinion, they are essential.

9.1 The Turing and the Mirror Test

At our conferences, which included topics such as artificial intelligence (AI), questions like "Does the SiMA model pass the Turing Test or even the Mirror Test?" continuously popped up. Such questions should be a thing of the past. To that end, it is important to know: These kinds of tests stem from a certain zeitgeist. They are based on knowledge and awareness of the time in which they were developed. They are based on observation of behavior. They are attempts to understand something with the knowledge of that time without having a *functional model*. Yet we know from physics, astronomy, chemistry, biology, and all the other natural sciences that real breakthroughs in all these subjects came only when they started to develop functional models stemming from observations of behavior. Tests such as the Turing Test or the Mirror Test, which were developed on the basis of a certain behavior, should therefore be viewed with reflection on their zeitgeist.

Let us start with the Turing Test. Alan Turing was a mathematician and is regarded as a pioneer of the theoretical (mathematical) foundations of computer and information theories. He did not have basic knowledge of psychoanalysis. He tried to understand the man-machine conflict from his point of view, from the point of view of a mathematician. This is, above all, the *language of logic*. What does thinking mean in this sense? Algorithms were his playing field. Put simply, algorithms can be seen as (mathematical) descriptions of the *behavior* of the flow of processes. However, we know from scientists like Wiener, Freud, or Braitenberg that in natural science the *functional* models have to be developed first. Of course, this development is based on the *behavior* model. Only by experimenting with these

D. Dietrich, *Artificial Intelligence: A Bridge Between Psychoanalysis and Neurology*, SpringerBriefs in Computer Science, https://doi.org/10.1007/978-3-031-30368-5_9

hypothetical functional models can a validation be achieved, which leads to a degree of certainty that the knowledge about an object can be regarded as correct. Nevertheless, as long as no experiment that proves that the hypotheses are wrong is found, the models may be assumed to be correct.

Mathematical models, on the other hand, are pure thought experiments and can not only be *validated* but also *proven*. The Turing test must be seen exactly from this point of view: It does not originate from any natural scientific reasoning. It is purely a mathematical (logically developed) thought model. Turing's [5] proposal of the *Imitation Game* as proof for human thinking is from today's point of view an outstanding pioneer work, but at the same time it has to be seen as a story from his zeitgeist. Today, scientists have to (axiomatically) define the terms *thinking*, *intelligence*, and *learning* more precisely, and do so in natural scientific terms. SiMA is a good example of this. It can be read from Fig. 8.5 that the definition of intelligence can be derived from the interaction of all the individual functions of the psyche or from the overall behavior of the Ψ-organ, depending on how the reference variables are determined. So there is no such thing as intelligence per se. Similar considerations apply to the notion of learning. But let us come back to Turing. Turing considered the process of communication between humans among themselves and humans and machines as a game of logic. For this reason, the term *test* is appropriate in the expression Turing Test. For mathematicians—and I have already addressed this topic—one can *test* a consideration or a logically formulated procedure, whether it is right or wrong. In natural science, on the other hand, it is better to speak of an *experiment*. In an experiment, there will always be deviations if one looks more closely at a physically or chemically based process. Therefore, the psychoanalyst today would design the experiment for identifying whether another human being or only a machine is sitting opposite the human being differently, in order to especially take into account the unconscious aspects of the communication between the subjects as well as the *transference* and the *countertransference* of a communication. Recognizing whether or not a machine is sitting opposite a human being depends on how detailed its Ψ-organ is structured and differentiated, how much information can be stored in it, how the parameters of the different functions are set, etc. One can then no longer speak of a test, only of an experiment that has to be validated. Proving no longer works. Real nature is involved. *To put it in a nutshell*: Turing juxtaposed a comparison of behavior. What is required, however, is a structural comparison (functional comparison) or a comparison in which at least a functional model of the Ψ-organ is placed on the side that is to be examined. *A machine developed via behavioral algorithms will never provide satisfactory results.*

Let us move on to the *Mirror Test*. Some years ago, scientists, for the first time, announced that their robots showed conscious behavior because they could recognize themselves in the mirror. What do these scientists intend with such absurd statements? Do they want to discredit psychologists? Do they want to attract attention?

The statements at least show how nonsensical it is to adopt findings, of a scientific field, from the past into the present time without any reflection—especially when findings from social science are applied one-to-one in natural science. The Mirror

Test is a behavioral test. It was developed at a time when people were not yet familiar with unconscious imaginations. There was no functional model of the psyche and especially not of the Ψ-organ. If you want to understand the Mirror Test today, you first have to adapt it to today's zeitgeist, to today's scientific knowledge. Without taking the unconscious information into account as well, the Mirror Test no longer makes sense today. If it is to be used at all in the scientific sense, then the axiomatics as well as a corresponding experiment must first be developed anew. There is no question that: Like the Turing Test, the Mirror Test in its former form must, from the psychoanalytic and scientific point of view, be regarded as obsolete.

9.2 Intelligence and Learning

Intelligence and learning ability can be attributed to each layer and each function in the Ψ-organ. A simple example: Intelligence and the ability to learn include the storage of information. In layer 1, the *learning ability* to store information means something different than in layer 2 or layer 3. In layer 1 (hardware), storing means the way information is physically stored. Neurologically speaking, we know two principles for this: interneuronal feedback, and storage via synapses. In layer 2 (neurosymbolism layer) and layer 3 (psyche), the storage of information is an associative principle, which can be relatively complex, especially if we think about the ways in which the information is accessed—regarding the connection to layer 1 over layer 2. Thus, storage in the Ψ-organ involves a complicated, multi-layered process. This has implications for learning and for intelligence. In dealing with the learning ability and intelligence of the layers and functions, one must define what exactly one wants to take into consideration. So far, science has dealt with learning and intelligence either too generally or with very specific principles, which in no case cover the complete and complex processes of the Ψ-organ.

I have to mention another point which is still hardly conceivable for some scientists. Chaotic discussions with colleagues have shown me this again and again. Up to now, the principle theorem in natural science that only experiments which are repeatable and thus clearly verifiable may be scientifically accepted was valid. This principle seemed to be set in stone. When a human being learns, and this also applies to technical information systems, he behaves differently after the learning process. *That is the meaning of a learning process.* The law that experiments must be reproducible, which seems to be set in stone, cannot apply to systems that are capable of learning. However, systems capable of learning are a part of scientific systems. Consider AI. Therefore, such a theorem which seems unalterable must be reconsidered. In SiMA, experiments of agents equipped with Ψ-organs are simulated. Their processes can still be repeated. However, if models like the SiMA model are fed with huge amounts of memories, this will no longer always be possible.

9.3 The Self

The *Self* is an "image" of the individual for the individual. It includes all sensory organs, not only the "visual", which shows that we ourselves still lack the right words for it. The Self is subjective. *It is always a picture of the past* and is constantly being overlaid with new information about how I "see" myself, how I feel. I can only guess at my earlier Self. The knowledge about it is constantly re-evaluated by my emotions and feelings. *Objectivity* about it from my point of view cannot exist, because all my thing and word representatives are constantly re-evaluated by myself through my recollection of them. This also means: *I continuously re-evaluate myself.* The Self is in constant flow.

The Self gives me knowledge about myself. Think of it as a large database of my psyche. It helps me to assess myself. It shows my current state—state of my psyche. It evaluates it. I get a sense of myself, which helps me behave in the way that seems optimal for me, wherever and however I move. I unconsciously move according to the defaults of my Self. Engineering has slowly understood that this ability is useful for complex machines. Modern airplanes are equipped with sensors and computers that continuously determine their own state in various situations so that the control systems can quickly and adequately react, and also plan for the long term.

Furthermore, the Self is the prerequisite for consciousness. If one wants to create an AI with consciousness, one must first figure out how the Self is to be integrated into the Ψ-organ of Fig. 8.5. In our team, Klaus Doblhammer, one of my colleagues in psychoanalysis, theoretically worked out the Self on the basis of psychoanalytic findings. It turned out that extensive programming work is necessary in order to be able to validate it experimentally in SiMA. An enormous amount of parameters have to be worked out and adjusted accordingly. Thus, up to now, his results could not be verified to a sufficient extent. This is a great pity, because only then does it make sense to deal with consciousness from a scientific point of view, which is the last big part in the modeling of the Ψ-organ.

Chapter 10
Scientific Elaboration of Consciousness

Consciousness has not yet been considered in the Ψ-Organ of the SiMA model. I just explained why. The first step must be to implement and validate the model concept of the Self. The next step is then to model the consciousness and validate it. The difficulty: Intensive discussions between computer engineers and psychoanalysts are still necessary on this path. Without this collaboration, little progress will be made, including designing the simulation experiments sensibly. The process requires clear axiomatics. But that is not all. Experiments in the natural sciences also require that they allow unambiguous interpretation and functional modeling [1, 9]. And we must be aware that we always formulate experiments from our current zeitgeist. Does the model of the Ψ-organ based on SiMA capture our zeitgeist? Have we overlooked certain aspects?

In principle, I do not see any insurmountable hurdles in integrating consciousness in the Ψ-organ and thus in our SiMA-agents. I also see no other way to understand the Ψ-organ on a scientific basis. And even if I am repeating myself: *We must make an effort to understand it, because it is the organ with which we try to understand.* Many believe algorithms are the solution. Yes! Algorithms are a powerful tool, without which we will not succeed in this endeavor. Algorithms are also the mainstay of SiMA. But they are only a mathematical tool, nothing more. However, the functional structure of the Ψ-organ is decisive. We have to work out all functions, just like physics works out its atomic model, like chemistry works out its model of the periodic table, and like neurology works out its neuronal network model.

Still, at conferences and in the scientific literature, I often sense a mood that I cannot understand: Many vehemently resist the *scientific elaboration of consciousness*. Many an author of today, many a film convey that artificial intelligence (AI) based on algorithms will surpass the abilities of humans, even make humans superfluous. Are we creating our own demise? Amazon, Facebook, and other AI-based systems whose algorithms know us better than we know ourselves are cited as examples. These algorithms make humans easier to manipulate. However, stop! Beware, these considerations involve two sets of issues. One is about the

D. Dietrich, *Artificial Intelligence: A Bridge Between Psychoanalysis and Neurology*, SpringerBriefs in Computer Science, https://doi.org/10.1007/978-3-031-30368-5_10

tools—the algorithms—that cause sociological and political difficulties. These dangerous components must always be observed. But this is unrelated to my request. What I would like to see in the development of the Ψ-organ and its simulation in order to test *our knowledge*, that is the second set of issues, is the inclusion of *consciousness*.

I associate the fear of dealing with consciousness from a scientific point of view with Freud's hint that mankind has had to endure three severe "blows of mankind" so far: the cosmological, the biological, and the psychological blow. The cosmological blow of mankind was the realization that our earth is not the center of the world. The biological (Darwinian) blow is the realization that man descended from the animal, and the third blow of mankind is the realization that "The ego is not master in its own house". The modeling of the Ψ-organ causes the fourth blow of the human being: *Thinking is not only reserved for humans and animals. We can enable machines to do it too.* That this is outrageous for many people is understandable to me. The fear of this must be overpowering. But SiMA speaks a clear language: *One can simulate and emulate the Ψ-organ.*

However, if we want to develop machines that autonomously save lives in dangerous areas, autonomously control drones for the transport of medicines, take over tasks from humans that are no longer reasonable for them, and can do these tasks better than humans, then these AI systems, these devices, must be given a (machine) consciousness. For this development, too, *we must learn to understand the Ψ-organ.* The ethical questions are questions of our zeitgeist. *We are forced to put them to the test.*

Literature (Cited in the Text)

1. Braitenberg, Valentin v.: Vehicles: Experiments in synthetic psychology. MIT Press, Cambridge; 1984
2. Damásio, A. R.: The Feeling of What Happens, Body and Emotion in the Making of Consciousness. Harcourt Brace & Company, New York; 1999
3. Damásio, A. R.: Looking for Spinoza; Joy, Sorrow and the Feeling Brain; William Heinemann : London; 2003
4. Dietrich, Dietmar.; Palensky, P.; Dietrich, Dorothee.: Psychoanalyse und Computertechnik eine Win-Win-Situation? psychosozial 35. Jg. (2012) Heft I (Nr. 127); S. 123-135.
5. Dietrich, D.; Jakubec, M.; Schaat, S.; Doblhammer, K.; Fodor, F.; Brandstätter, Chr.: The Fourth Outrage of Man – Is the Turing-test Still Up to Date? Journal of Computers, Vol. 12, Nr. 2, S. 116 – 126; 2017
6. Dietrich, D.: Simulating the Mind II, Forschungsergebnisse, Psychoanalyse, Neurologie, Künstliche Intelligenz: ein Modell. Shaker Verlag; 2021
7. Hawkins, J.: On Intelligence. Henry Holt and Company, New York, 2004
8. Gabbard, Glen O. ; Litowitz, Bonnie E.; Williams, Paul: Textbook of Psychoanalysis, Second Edition, American Psychiatric Publishing; 2012
9. Luria, A. R.: The Working Brain, An Introduction to Neuropsychology; Basic Books, A Member of the Perseus Books Group; 1973
10. Palensky, B.: Introducing Neuro-Psychoanalysis towards the Design of Cognitive and Affective Automation Systems; Ph.D. thesis at the Institute of Computer Technology, Technische Universität Wien (Austria); 2008
11. Peterfreund, E.; Schwartz, J.: Information, systems, and psychoanalysis. An evolutionary biological approach to psychoanalytic theory. New York: International University Press; 1971
12. Sloman, A.: Machines in the Ghost; in: Simulating the Mind, A Technical Neuropsychoanalytical Approach; Editors: Dietmar Dietrich, Georg Fodor, Gerhard Zucker, Dietmar Bruckner, Springer Wien New York; 2009
13. Solms, M., Turnbull, O.: The Brain and the Inner World. An introduction to the neuroscience of subjective experience. Karnac/Other Press, represented by Cathy Miller Foreign Rights Agency, London, England; 2002
14. Turkle, Sh.: Artificial Intelligence and Psychoanalysis: A New Alliance; in the Artificial Intelligence Debate; False Starts, Real Foundations; Edited by Stephen R. Graubard; MIT Press; 1988; S. 242–268
15. Yoram, Y.: Return of the Zombie – Neuropsychoanalysis, Consciousness, and the Engineering of Psychic Functions; in: Simulating the Mind, A Technical Neuropsychoanalytical Approach;

© The Author(s), under exclusive license to Springer Nature Switzerland AG 2023
D. Dietrich, *Artificial Intelligence: A Bridge Between Psychoanalysis and Neurology*, SpringerBriefs in Computer Science,
https://doi.org/10.1007/978-3-031-30368-5

Editors: Dietmar Dietrich, Georg Fodor, Gerhard Zucker, Dietmar Bruckner, Springer Wien New York; 2009

Several Bibliographic Notes

To [1]—Braitenberg succeeds in making it easy for the reader to understand and describe an object from the point of view of its function on the one hand, and its behavior on the other.

To [2]—Damasió does not use a term like Ψ-organ, but he sees his exact task in understanding this as a unified organ, in which concepts like affects, emotions, feelings or consciousness have to be worked out axiomatically from a natural scientific point of view.

To [4]—Marianne Leuzinger-Bohleber is a highly respected scholar of psychoanalysis. Her list of publications is very impressive. However, the essay listed here shows that even such scientists can quickly go astray when they try to understand the worlds of natural and information science with the methods of their world (hermeneutics).

To [5]—The article dispels the illusion that phenomena to be explained psychologically or psychoanalytically can be understood (worked out) purely logically. It requires knowledge of the experiments of psychology or psychoanalysis, but it shows the genius of Turing.

To [6]—The first book, "Simulating the Mind", was written together with international scientists and is therefore written in English. Dietrich wrote the second book without other authors. The contents are the results of the SiMA project (Simulating of the Mental Apparatus & Applications), on which many scientists worked for more than 20 years.

To [7]—Jeff Hawkins is the inventor of the Palm Pilot and co-founder of Palm Inc. as well as a neuroscientist (Redwood Neuroscience Institute). He sold his company and used the proceeds to work on one topic in particular: How to model the brain. He came across unbelievable findings over his decades of research.

To [8]—The textbook is comprehensive and provides insight into various orientations such as those of Klein, Bion, and Lacan.

To [10]—Damásio knows how to uniquely explain that feeling and thinking, from a scientific point of view, cannot be considered separately. For me, however, the book has an additional essential meaning: He finds the connection to Spinoza in this context. However, unlike Leibniz, Goethe, Newton, Einstein and many others who were also deeply impressed by Spinoza, Damásio did not shy away from addressing him at length in this book of his.

To [11]—The dissertation excellently reflects various model ideas of artificial intelligence relevant to SiMA.

To [13]—The two scientists manage to introduce the reader to the neurological and psychoanalytical worlds of our thinking system in a language that even non-experts can understand.

Index

A

Abstract, 3, 23, 38
Act, 44
Actuator, 2
Affect, X
Affect, quota of, X, 27, 30, 42
Agent, 26
Aggressive, 42
AIBO ERS-7M§, 26
Algorithms, 47, 51
Analog, 9, 20
AND, 9
Anger, 30, 42
Animal, 16
Apparatus, mental, 1
Artificial intelligence (AI), 26, 51
Associate, 33
Associative abilities, 30
Aware, 32
Axiomatic, X, 5, 6
Axon, 19

B

Bees, 15
Behavior, 7, 21, 26, 47
Behavioral phenomena, 8, 26
Behavior, human, 26
Big bang, 11
Binary, 9
Binary logic, 20
Black box, 39
Blows of mankind, 52
Body, 29

Body perception track, 40
Body, human, 16
Bottom-up method, 16, 20
Brain, 1, 2, 15
Brainstorming, 30
Braitenberg, Valentin von, 7
Breast, 33, 41, 43

C

Camera system, 26
Capability, 24
Carriers of information, 19
Cat, 32
Cathexis, 27
Causality, 45
Cerebellum, 21
Cerebrum, 21
Certain proximity, 4
Charge carriers, 20
Chemistry, 3
Circuits, digital, 12
Clock, 3
Coding, 23, 36
Communication, 15
Completeness, 8
Complexity, 7
Computer, biological, 16
Computer, quantum, 20
Computers, 19
Conflict, 29
Conflict resolution, 31
Conscious, 4, 32
Conscious information, 31

Consciously, 38
Consciousness, 31, 43, 50
Consciousness, machine, 52
Contradiction, 4, 5, 29
Contrast, 24
Control engineering, 5
Coupling of the functions, 21
Culture, 5
Cup, 23
Cyberneticist, 7

D
Darwin, Charles, 52
Decimal, 9
Decision, 29, 31
Decoding, 25, 36
Defense, 30, 33
Defense track, 43
Definitions of terms, 5
Delay time, 11
Dendrite, 19
Describe, 3
Description language, 20
Desexualization, 42
Design, 15, 20
Design language, 12
Desymbolization, 25
Digital, 20
Discharging, 19
Displacement, 41, 43
Dog, 32
Dream, 30
Drive, 42
Drive source, 29
Drive target, 29
Drive track, 28, 29, 41
Drive wish, 41
Dummy, 38
Dynamic, 29

E
Economic, 29
Ego, 27
Emotion, 27, 30, 42
Emotion, basic, 30
Emotion, extended, 30
Energy, physical, 30
Energy, psychic, 30
Environment track, 40
Envy, 30
Evaluation, 42

Experiment, 1, 4, 5, 12, 49
Eye, 26

F
Fear, 30, 42
Feedback, 21, 44
Feeling, 30, 42
Fire, 19
Fly, 32
Forgetting, 33
Freud, 8, 25
Function, 6, 7, 11, 26
Future, 30, 32, 44

G
Greed, 30

H
Handicraft, 20
Happiness elation, 42
Happiness saturation, 42
Hardware, 13
Hardware function, 21
Hawking, Stephen, 11
Hawkins, Jeff, 25, 40
Heisenberg, Werner, 4
Holistic, 1
Homeostasis, 27, 29, 41
Hormonal system, 21
Hormone, 29
Hubris, 25
Humanities, 3, 5
Hunger, 41, 43
Hypotheses, 48

I
Id, 27
Impulse, 35
Information, 2, 3, 5
Information channels, 21
Information, conflicting, 29
Information, conscious, 31
Information processing laws, 20
Information symbols, 23
Information system, 1, 8, 35
Information theory, 9, 15
Intelligence, 15, 48
Intelligence, active, 15
Intelligence, structural, 15

Intensity, psychic, 30
Interdependency, structural, 39
Interface, 9, 11, 21, 23, 36
Internet of Things, 5
ISO/OSI, 12, 16

J
Joy, 30, 42

K
Kandel, Eric, 32

L
L2, L3, 35
Language, description, 20
Layer, 38
Learning, 48, 49
Level, 38
Libidinous, 42
Logic, 2, 4, 5, 31, 47
Logic, temporal, causal, 30

M
Mathematics, 2, 4
Matter, 3
Mealy, 2, 3, 11, 16, 27
Mealy machine, 12
Memory, 29
Memory, long-term, 21
Memory, short-term, 21
Metapsychology, 8
Method, 3, 29
Method, description, 11
Methods, clinical, 27
Mirror Test, 47, 48
Model, 3
Model, behavior, 2, 16, 27
Model, data, 27
Model, functional, 2, 16
Model, layer, 11
Model, second topographical, 16
Model, structural, 16
Model, three-layer, 23
Model, topographical, 8, 27
Monkey, 32
Mother's breast, 33
Multi-value logic, 9

N
Natural sciences, 3, 42
Nerve, 9, 17
Nervous system, 2, 15
Network, neuronal, 19
Neural network, 19, 23
Neurology, 5, 27
Neuron, 9, 15, 17, 19, 32
Neuroscience, 26
Neurosymbolic layer, 23
Neurosymbolism, 24
Neurosymbolization, 36
Neurotransmitters, 19
Nonlinear, 19

O
Objectivity, 1, 4, 33
Oral, 33
Organ, 2
Organ, nervous, 16
OSI, 12

P
Past, 32, 44
Perception, 25
Perception track, 29, 40
Perception, neutral, 28
Philosophy, 1, 5
Physical energy, 21
Physics, 3
Plan, 30, 44
Pleasure, 30, 41
Pride, 30
Primary process, 27, 39
Probability, 4
Process, 15
Processing, 15
Project, 31
Proving, 4
Ψ-organ, 2, 15, 20, 21
Psyche, 1, 2, 5, 15
Psychic apparatus, 2
Psychic intensity, 30, 41
Psychoanalysis, 2, 5
Psychoanalysis, advantage of, 27
Psychology, 2, 8
Pulse, 11
Pulse width, 20

Q
Quota of affect, X, 27, 29, 30, 42

R
Reality, 23, 45
Reductionism, neurological, 2
Reference, 1
Religion, 1, 5
Repeatability, 49
Representative, 9, 23, 28, 35, 36
Representative regression, 36
Representatives, valued, 32
Repressed, primally, 41
Repression, primal, 33
Reproduction, 42
Rule, 30
Rules, internalized, 30

S
Sadness, 42
Secondary process, 27, 44
Self, 32, 50
Self-preservation, 28
Self-preservation drive representatives, 41
Sensor, 7
Sex drive representative, 41
Sexual drive, 28
Signals, electrical, 23
SiMA, 5, 23
Simulation, 2, 26
Singularity, 11
Social environment, 30
Sony, 26
Spinoza, Baruch, 1
Spirit, 1
Standardization bodies, 5
Storage, 15, 21, 32
Storage process, 32
Strategies, 30
Structure, 7, 21
Subjective, 30, 50
Sublimation, 41, 42
Supercomputer, 20
Superego, 27, 43
Superego, proactive, reactive, 30
Suppress, 31
Symbol, 23, 35, 36
Symbol Grounding, 32
Symbolically, 21
Symbolic quantities, 21

Symbol production, 35
Synapse, 19, 21, 32
Synthesis, 20

T
Ternary, 9, 20
Test, 47
Thing representative, 28, 30
Thinking, 48
Thinking apparatus, 1
3D model, 39
Threshold, 19
Threshold logic, 20
Tool, 4, 51
Top-down method, 16
Topographical, 29
Track, 40
Track, action decision, 45
Track, defense, 45
Track, desire and need selection, 45
Trades, 5
Trial actions, 31, 45
Turing Test, 47

U
Uncertainty principle, 4
Unconscious, 16
Unpleasure, 30, 41

V
Validating, 4
Validation, 48
Vehicles, 7

W
Wiener, Norbert, 44
Willfully, 38
Word assignment, 32
Word representative, 28
World, inner, 24
World, outer, 24
Worm, 32

Z
Zeitgeist, 1, 5, 42, 47